Cultivating Mindfulness, Self-Awareness and Growth

7 Exercises for Living a More Fulfilling Life

by

Yolanda Trevino

First Edition

Lightbody Publishing

P.O. Box 151 Lafayette, CA, USA

Copyright © 2023 by Yolanda Trevino. All rights reserved.

Published by Lightbody Publishing, LLC

P.O. Box 151

Lafayette, CA 94549

www.lightbodypublishing.com

First Edition: August 8, 2023

ISBN: 978-1-7371595-2-0

All rights reserved. No part of this publication may be reproduced, distributed, or transmitted in any form or by any means, including photocopying, recording, or other electronic or mechanical methods, without the prior written permission of the publisher, except in the case of brief quotations embodied in critical reviews and certain other noncommercial uses permitted by copyright law.

This book is designed to provide general information on the topics presented. It is not intended to be a substitute for professional advice or treatment, and the author and publisher expressly disclaim any and all liability arising directly or indirectly from the use of this book.

Please consult a qualified professional regarding your specific needs and circumstances before making any decisions or taking any actions based on the information in this book.

By purchasing and reading this book, you acknowledge that you have read and understood the above information and agree to be bound by the terms and conditions stated herein.

Disclaimer

The information in this book is provided for general informational and educational purposes only and is not a substitute for professional advice. The author and publisher are not responsible for any actions or inaction on your part based on the information presented in this book. The exercises and practices presented in this book may not be suitable for everyone, and it is recommended that you consult with a professional before beginning any new exercise or wellness program. The author and publisher make no representations or warranties with respect to the accuracy, applicability, fitness, or completeness of the contents of this book. The author and publisher disclaim any warranties (express or implied), merchantability, or fitness for any particular purpose. The author and publisher shall in no event be held liable to any party for any direct, indirect, punitive, special, incidental or other consequential damages arising directly or indirectly from any use of this material, which is provided 'as is', and without warranties."

Dedication

To those who have felt discouraged or held back by the unsupportive people in their lives, may this book serve as a reminder that you have the power within you to overcome obstacles, transform yourself, and live a fulfilling life. Keep pushing forward and never give up on your dreams! This book is dedicated to you.

About Author

Yolanda Trevino is a writer, entrepreneur, and coach dedicated to helping individuals achieve personal growth and transformation. She is the founder of Evolutionary Body System, a self-discovery program designed to empower individuals to unlock their full potential and achieve a greater sense of well-being.

Yolanda's passion for personal growth and development began in the beauty industry, where she recognized the profound significance of self-care and self-love. Her experiences inspired her to explore other areas of personal growth and development, leading her to write three books under her publishing company, Lightbody Publishing, LLC. Her latest book, "Cultivating Mindfulness, Self-Awareness and Growth: 7 Exercises for Living a More Fulfilling Life," offers practical exercises and insights for personal growth and self-improvement.

In addition to her latest book, Yolanda is also the author of "What's in Emerald City: The Power of the Heart," a powerful memoir that courageously explores the impact of various types of trauma. This deeply personal work sheds light on the human spirit's resilience and the healing power of love and self-discovery.

Her second book, "Lessons Learned at 40 - A Journey of Growth and Self-Discovery," is a collection of personal essays that offer practical advice and inspiration to help readers achieve their goals and embrace personal growth.

As a sought-after speaker, Yolanda shares her insights and experiences with audiences around the world. She is also an advocate for health and wellness, exploring the benefits of clean eating and staying active through gym workouts and nature walks. Yolanda is a lifelong learner and is actively involved in volunteering and giving back to her community.

Yolanda resides in the San Francisco Bay Area, where she continues to pursue her passions with unwavering dedication and determination.

Table of Contents

Introduction 1

1. Self-Reflection And Self-Love 3
2. Visualization 26
3. Cultivating Healthy Relationships (Building Support System/Emotional Intelligence) 38
4. Nutrition And Fitness 51
5. Developing A Growth Mindset And Resilience 66
6. Creating Healthy Habits And Self-Care 80
7. Meditation/Mindfulness 91

Conclusion 107

7 Exercises For Living A More Fulfilling Life 109

Acknowledgments 115

References And Web Links 116

Introduction

Welcome to "7 Exercises for Living a More Fulfilling Life." This book represents the culmination of years of personal growth and transformation in my life, inspired by my experiences and the lessons I learned during my journey of growth and self-discovery. This includes the development of my program, the Evolutionary Body System, which is based on the idea that we all have the capacity to evolve and transform ourselves, regardless of where we are in life. As I was finishing my book, "Lessons Learned at 40: A Journey of Growth and Self-Discovery," I developed a set of exercises that were inspired by the techniques and practices in my program, and had helped me achieve a greater sense of fulfillment and well-being.

One of the key lessons that I've learned along my own path is that the only way to truly let go of the past and overcome our challenges is to face them directly. It took me years to learn this, and I'm excited to share the blueprint with you that helped me transform my own life, so you can overcome your own challenges as soon as possible, as long as you're willing to put in the work. The exercises in this book are a distillation of the tools, techniques, and practices that I used, and I'm thrilled to share them with you.

The order of the sections in this book was carefully crafted to provide a gradual path towards personal growth, starting with the basics of self-care and self-love, which form the foundation for all the exercises and practices that follow. From there, the book builds up to more complex techniques and knowledge, guiding you on a journey towards cultivating a positive relationship with yourself, setting clear goals, developing healthy relationships, improving your physical and mental health, overcoming obstacles, and creating a daily self-care routine.

Remember that personal growth is a lifelong journey, and it requires patience, commitment, and the willingness to step outside of our comfort zones. However, I believe that you have the power within you to create the life you want, and this book is here to support and guide you every step of the way. So let's get started on this transformative journey together with the 7 exercises presented in this book.

Self-reflection and self-love

INTRODUCTION OVERVIEW: The first section of this book sets the foundation for personal growth and well-being by exploring the fundamental concepts of self-awareness and self-love. Self-awareness is the ability to recognize our thoughts, emotions, and behaviors and understand how they impact our lives. Self-love, on the other hand, is about cultivating a positive relationship with ourselves, accepting who we are, and treating ourselves with kindness and compassion.

This section delves into why self-awareness and self-love are essential components of personal growth. It will discuss how they relate to each other and why they are crucial for developing a more fulfilling and meaningful life. By practicing self-awareness, we can identify negative patterns and behaviors that may be holding us back and make positive changes in our lives. By cultivating self-love, we can develop a positive self-image, increase self-confidence, and improve our relationships with others.

The importance of self-awareness and self-love cannot be overstated. Without self-awareness, we may struggle to identify and address our own needs and desires, and without self-love, we may find it challenging to form positive relationships with others. By developing both, we can create a strong foundation for personal growth and well-being.

In addition to discussing the importance of self-awareness and self-love, this section will provide actionable tips and techniques for cultivating these qualities in your daily life. Journaling, meditation, and other self-reflection exercises can be incredibly effective in developing self-awareness and self-love. By practicing these techniques, you can gain a deeper understanding of your thoughts and emotions, challenge negative self-talk, and develop greater self-compassion.

In summary, the first section of this book emphasizes the importance of self-awareness and self-love for personal growth and well-being. By cultivating these qualities in our daily lives, we can gain a deeper understanding of ourselves, form more positive relationships with others, and lead a more fulfilling and meaningful life. Through practical tips and techniques, this section provides actionable steps to help readers develop self-awareness and self-love.

- **Understanding the importance of self-awareness and self-love for personal growth and well-being:**

Self-awareness and self-love are crucial for personal growth and well-being. Individuals who cultivate these practices in their lives often experience a wide range of benefits. For instance, self-awareness can help individuals develop a deeper understanding of their thoughts, emotions, and behaviors. By becoming more aware of their inner experiences, individuals can learn to regulate their emotions and respond to situations in a more thoughtful and effective manner. This improved emotional regulation can lead to a greater sense of calm, decreased stress and anxiety, and improved overall well-being.

Self-love, on the other hand, involves developing a positive relationship with oneself. By cultivating self-love, individuals can learn to treat themselves with kindness, compassion, and understanding. This can lead to greater self-esteem, improved confidence, and an increased sense of self-worth. Individuals who practice self-love may also experience more fulfilling relationships, as they are able to approach their interactions with others from a place of self-respect and confidence.

Research and studies have shown that self-awareness and self-love are associated with a range of positive outcomes. For example, one study found that individuals with higher levels of self-awareness were more likely to experience improved relationships, better decision-making, and increased job satisfaction. Another study found that self-love was associated with decreased stress and improved overall mental health. [1, 2, 3, 4]

Meet Jane, a successful entrepreneur and single mother of three, struggled with self-doubt and imposter syndrome for years. She found herself constantly seeking validation from others and neglecting her own needs, leading to feelings of burnout and unhappiness. However, after beginning a daily practice of journaling and meditation, Jane discovered the power of self-reflection and self-love in transforming her life.

By identifying and challenging her limiting beliefs, Jane was able to cultivate a growth mindset and a greater sense of self-compassion. She learned to set healthy boundaries and prioritize her own well-being, resulting in improved emotional regulation, greater clarity and direction in life, and more fulfilling relationships. With the help of a coach, she was able to gain deeper insights into her patterns and behaviors and create lasting change in her life.

Jane's story is just one example of how the practices of self-awareness and self-love can lead to transformative personal growth and fulfillment. Many others have also applied these practices to their lives with great success.

And there's Robert, a 32-year-old software engineer who had been struggling with anxiety and stress for years. Robert had always been a high achiever, pushing himself to succeed in his career and personal life. However, this drive had taken a toll on his mental and emotional health. He found himself constantly worrying about work, relationships, and his future.

Through a period of self-reflection, Robert began to realize that he had been neglecting his own needs and placing too much emphasis on external validation. He decided to make changes in his life to prioritize his own well-being. He began practicing mindfulness and meditation to reduce stress and anxiety, and took up yoga to improve his physical health.

With these practices in place, Robert began to develop greater self-awareness and a more positive self-image. He learned to set healthy boundaries and prioritize his own needs, leading to more fulfilling relationships with friends and family. As he became more confident in his own abilities and more compassionate toward himself, he found that his anxiety and stress levels began to decrease.

Research has shown that practices such as mindfulness, meditation, and self-compassion can have a positive impact on mental and emotional health.[5, 6, 7, 8] Robert is a living example of the benefits of self-awareness and self-love. Through his own personal journey, he has found greater fulfillment and joy in his life.

Self-love involves treating oneself with kindness, compassion, and understanding, and cultivating a positive relationship with oneself. When individuals practice self-love, they are able to approach their interactions with others from a place of self-respect and confidence. This can lead to more fulfilling relationships, as they are able to set healthy boundaries, communicate their needs, and approach conflicts with a sense of self-assurance.

Additionally, practicing self-love can improve self-esteem and confidence. By cultivating self-compassion and positive self-talk, individuals can learn to appreciate their strengths and abilities, and approach challenges with a growth mindset. This can lead to greater confidence and a sense of self-worth, which can positively impact all areas of life.

In summary, the subtopics under "Self-reflection and self-love" are crucial for personal growth and well-being. These include understanding the importance of self-awareness and self-love, practicing self-reflection, identifying limiting beliefs and patterns, cultivating self-compassion and positive self-talk, learning to set healthy boundaries and prioritize needs, and exploring self-care practices. By engaging in these practices, individuals can improve their emotional resilience, gain clarity and direction in life, and experience greater self-esteem, confidence, and fulfilling relationships.

Now, try thinking of some simple and practical techniques you can begin implementing into your daily life now. Perhaps you can start by setting aside some time each day for self-reflection and journaling, or by trying out a guided meditation practice to improve emotional regulation. Whatever techniques you choose, the key is to make them a regular part of your routine and approach them with a sense of curiosity and openness.

Remember, the journey toward greater self-awareness and self-love is a lifelong process. Each new technique or insight you gain builds upon the last, creating a solid foundation for ongoing growth and personal fulfillment that will support you in all areas of your life.

- **Practicing self-reflection through journaling, meditation, or quiet contemplation:**

Practicing self-reflection is an essential tool for personal growth and self-awareness. It is a deliberate practice of taking the time to reflect on our thoughts, emotions, and behaviors, in order to gain deeper insights into ourselves and our experiences. There are several effective techniques for practicing self-reflection, but journaling, meditation, and quiet contemplation are three of the most popular and effective techniques.

Journaling involves putting your thoughts and feelings down on paper, while meditation involves focusing your attention on your breath or a particular object. Quiet contemplation involves setting aside time to reflect on your thoughts and experiences without any distractions.

The benefits of practicing self-reflection through journaling, meditation, or quiet contemplation are numerous. Self-reflection can help individuals identify and challenge negative thought patterns, gain greater clarity and insight into their experiences, and develop a deeper sense of self-awareness. It can also lead to increased emotional regulation, decreased stress and anxiety, and improved overall well-being.

To get started with self-reflection, it can be helpful to set aside a dedicated time and space for it. This can be a specific time of day or a particular location that helps you feel relaxed and focused. It is also important to approach self-reflection with an open and non-judgmental attitude, allowing yourself to explore your thoughts and feelings without fear of judgment or criticism.

Consider the story of Jill, a 35-year-old teacher and mother of two who struggled with feelings of stress and overwhelm in her daily life. She found herself constantly worrying about her work, her relationships, and her future. However, after starting a daily journaling practice, Jill discovered the power of self-reflection in helping her gain greater clarity and insight into her experiences.

Through her journaling practice, Jill was able to identify and challenge negative thought patterns and develop a deeper sense of self-awareness. She found that taking the time to reflect on her thoughts and feelings helped her gain a greater sense of control over her life and feel more grounded and centered.

Research and studies have shown that self-reflection practices such as journaling, meditation, and quiet contemplation can have a positive impact on mental and emotional well-being. For instance, one study found that individuals who practice self-reflection experience decreased levels of stress and anxiety, improved self-awareness, and increased emotional regulation. [9, 10, 11]

In summary, self-reflection is a powerful tool for personal growth and self-awareness. By practicing self-reflection through journaling, meditation, or quiet contemplation, individuals can gain greater clarity and insight into their experiences, identify and challenge negative thought patterns, and improve their overall well-being. We'll explore meditation and techniques for meditation later in the book. For now, to get started with self-reflection, set aside a dedicated time and space for reflection, approach self-reflection with an open and non-judgmental attitude, and experiment with different techniques to find what works best for you. Remember, the journey toward greater self-awareness and self-love is a lifelong process. Each new insight and technique you gain builds upon the last, creating a solid foundation for ongoing growth and personal fulfillment that will support you in all areas of your life.

- **Identifying limiting beliefs and patterns that may be holding you back**

Identifying limiting beliefs and patterns that may be holding you back is an essential step in the journey of personal growth and self-awareness. Limiting beliefs are negative or self-defeating thoughts that can prevent us from realizing our full potential. These beliefs can be deeply ingrained in our minds, often stemming from past experiences, societal conditioning, or other external factors.

The first step in identifying limiting beliefs and patterns is to become aware of them. This can involve paying attention to our self-talk and noticing when negative or self-defeating thoughts arise. It can also involve reflecting on past experiences and the messages we received about ourselves from others.

Once we have identified our limiting beliefs and patterns, we can begin to challenge them. This involves questioning the validity of these beliefs and considering alternative perspectives. We can also look for evidence that contradicts these beliefs and identify ways in which they may be holding us back.

By identifying and challenging our limiting beliefs and patterns, we can develop a growth mindset and open ourselves up to new opportunities and experiences. We can also gain a greater sense of self-awareness and self-acceptance, which can lead to improved emotional regulation and more fulfilling relationships.

Let's take a look at an example to illustrate this. Meet Maya, a 30-year-old artist who struggled with self-doubt and imposter syndrome for years. Maya had always been passionate about art, but her fear of failure and criticism held her back from pursuing it professionally. After recognizing her limiting beliefs and patterns through therapy, Maya began to challenge her beliefs and question her assumptions. She reframed her perspective and started pursuing her passion, eventually becoming a successful artist.

Through self-reflection and therapy, May was able to identify the limiting beliefs and patterns that were holding her back. She discovered that many of these beliefs were rooted in her fear of failure and a need

Cultivating Mindfulness, Self-Awareness and Growth

for perfectionism. By challenging these beliefs and reframing her perspective, May was able to overcome her self-doubt and take bold steps in her career and personal life.

Sally's story is another example of how limiting beliefs and patterns can hold us back. Sally, a 25-year-old recent college graduate who was struggling to find a job in her field. Sally had always been told by her parents that she wasn't good enough and that she would never be successful. These beliefs had been deeply ingrained in her mind, and she found herself feeling anxious and defeated in her job search.

Through self-reflection and journaling, Sally was able to identify the limiting beliefs that were holding her back. She realized that she had been internalizing her parents' negative attitudes toward her and that this was causing her to doubt her own abilities. Sally became aware that her parents' attitudes towards her were not a reflection of her abilities, but rather their own internal problems. By challenging these beliefs and replacing them with more positive and empowering thoughts, Sally felt more confident and capable. She was eventually able to secure a job in her field.

Research and studies have shown that identifying and challenging limiting beliefs and patterns can have a positive impact on mental and emotional health. For example, a study found that cognitive behavioral therapy, which involves identifying and challenging negative thought patterns, can lead to improved symptoms of depression and anxiety. [12, 13, 14]

To begin identifying and challenging your own limiting beliefs and patterns, start by paying attention to your self-talk and reflecting on past experiences. Ask yourself what beliefs may be holding you back, and consider alternative perspectives. Look for evidence that contradicts your limiting beliefs and identify ways in which they may be preventing you from realizing your full potential.

In summary, identifying limiting beliefs and patterns that may be holding you back is an important step in personal growth and self-awareness. By becoming aware of these beliefs and patterns, we can challenge them and develop a growth mindset, which can lead to greater self-awareness and self-acceptance, improved emotional regulation, and more fulfilling relationships.

- **Cultivating self-compassion and positive self-talk**

Cultivating self-compassion and positive self-talk is essential for improving one's overall well-being and mental health. When individuals are able to treat themselves with kindness, compassion, and understanding, they are better equipped to cope with the challenges and stresses of life. This subtopic will explore what self-compassion and positive self-talk are, why they are important, and how individuals can cultivate these practices in their daily lives.

Self-compassion involves treating oneself with the same level of kindness, concern, and understanding that one would offer to a close friend or loved one. By extending this same level of compassion to oneself, individuals can begin to develop a more positive self-image and greater emotional resilience. Positive self-talk is a way to reinforce this self-compassion by intentionally choosing to speak to oneself in a supportive and uplifting manner.

Research has shown that practicing self-compassion and positive self-talk can lead to a range of positive outcomes, including improved self-esteem, reduced stress and anxiety, and improved overall well-being. For example, one study found that individuals who practiced self-compassion were less likely to experience symptoms of depression and anxiety. [15, 16, 17, 18]

One way to cultivate self-compassion and positive self-talk is through mindfulness practices such as meditation and deep breathing. These practices can help individuals become more aware of their thoughts and emotions and learn to approach them with kindness and understanding. Additionally, individuals can begin to challenge negative self-talk and replace it with positive affirmations and thoughts.

Take the example of Alice, a 26-year-old dental assistant who struggled with self-doubt and feelings of inadequacy. She found herself constantly comparing herself to others and focusing on her flaws and shortcomings. However, with the help of a therapist, Alice learned to identify and challenge her negative self-talk and cultivate self-compassion.

Through mindfulness practices such as meditation and deep breathing, Alice was able to become more aware of her thoughts and emotions and approach them with kindness and understanding. She also began to challenge her negative self-talk and replace it with positive affirmations and thoughts. Over time, Alice noticed that her self-esteem improved, and she was better able to cope with the stresses of her job and personal life.

Now, meet David, a 40-year-old business executive and father of three. David had always been a high achiever, but he found himself struggling with feelings of self-doubt and inadequacy. He often felt like he wasn't doing enough, or that he wasn't living up to his own expectations.

Through a period of self-reflection, David realized that his negative self-talk was holding him back from reaching his full potential. He decided to start practicing self-compassion and positive self-talk. He began by identifying his negative self-talk patterns and replacing them with positive affirmations and compassionate statements. He also started a daily gratitude practice to focus on the positive aspects of his life.

As he continued to practice self-compassion and positive self-talk, David noticed a significant shift in his mindset. He began to feel more confident in his abilities and less critical of himself. He found that he was able to approach his work and personal life with greater ease and enjoyment. He also found that his relationships with his family and colleagues improved, as he was able to communicate his needs and boundaries more effectively.

These two stories illustrate the power of self-compassion and positive self-talk in transforming one's mindset and approach to life. By cultivating a kind and compassionate relationship with oneself, individuals can improve their emotional well-being, boost their confidence and self-esteem, and create more fulfilling relationships with others.

Cultivating self-compassion and positive self-talk is an essential component of personal growth and well-being. By treating oneself with kindness, compassion, and understanding, individuals can improve their overall mental health and well-being. Mindfulness practices such as meditation and deep breathing can help individuals become more aware of their thoughts and emotions and learn to approach them with kindness and understanding. Additionally, individuals can begin to challenge negative self-talk and replace it with positive affirmations and thoughts.

To put these concepts into action, readers are encouraged to start by becoming more aware of their inner self-talk and begin to challenge negative self-talk with positive affirmations and thoughts. By practicing mindfulness and other self-compassion techniques, individuals can cultivate a more positive self-image and greater emotional resilience in their daily lives.

- **Learning to set healthy boundaries and prioritize your needs:**

Learning to set healthy boundaries and prioritize your needs is an essential component of self-care and self-love. Many of us struggle with saying "no" to others or taking on too much, which can lead to burnout, stress, and even resentment. By learning to set healthy boundaries and prioritize our own needs, we can create a more balanced and fulfilling life.

One example of the importance of setting healthy boundaries comes from the story of Naya, a 35-year-old marketing executive. Naya had always been a people pleaser, saying "yes" to every request that came her way, even if it meant sacrificing her own needs and well-being. She found herself feeling drained and overwhelmed, and her work and relationships began to suffer.

After some self-reflection and guidance from a therapist, Naya learned to set healthy boundaries with others. She started saying "no" to requests that didn't align with her priorities, and made sure to prioritize her own self-care and well-being. As a result, she experienced greater energy and focus in her work, and deeper, more meaningful relationships with her friends and family.

To cultivate healthy boundaries in your own life, it's important to start by identifying what your own needs and priorities are. What activities, relationships, or tasks are most important to you, and how can you make sure to prioritize them in your life? Once you've identified your priorities, practice saying "no" to requests that don't align with them. Remember that it's okay to prioritize your own well-being, and that saying "no" to others is not a reflection of your worth.

In addition to setting boundaries with others, it's also important to set boundaries with ourselves. This means being mindful of our own self-talk and avoiding negative self-judgments or unrealistic expectations. Cultivating self-compassion and positive self-talk can help us be kinder and more patient with ourselves, which can lead to greater confidence and self-esteem.

To start setting healthy boundaries and prioritizing your needs, try some of the following tips and techniques:

- Identify your priorities and make sure to schedule time for them in your life

- Practice saying "no" to requests that don't align with your priorities

- Avoid negative self-talk and practice self-compassion and positive self-talk

- Seek support from a therapist, coach, or trusted friend or family member

In summary, learning to set healthy boundaries and prioritize your needs is an essential component of self-care and self-love. By identifying your priorities and practicing saying "no" to requests that don't align with them, you can create a more balanced and fulfilling life. Remember to also set boundaries with yourself, and practice self-compassion and positive self-talk to improve your confidence and self-esteem.

- **Exploring practices for self-care and self-love**

Self-care and self-love are important components of overall well-being. Taking care of ourselves physically, emotionally, and mentally can help us cultivate a greater sense of self-compassion, reduce stress and anxiety, and improve our overall health. In this section, we will explore some of the practices and techniques that can help individuals develop self-care and self-love in their daily lives.

Self-care and self-love involve taking care of oneself and cultivating a positive relationship with oneself. Self-care practices may include things like exercise, healthy eating, getting enough sleep, and engaging in activities that bring joy and relaxation. Self-love practices involve developing a sense of self-compassion and positive self-talk, which can lead to increased self-esteem and greater confidence.

Meet Sandra, a 40-year-old accountant and mother of two. For years, Sandra had been neglecting her own needs, focusing instead on her job and her children. She found herself feeling drained and unhappy, with little energy or enthusiasm for life.

Through self-reflection and exploration, Sandra began to realize the importance of self-care and self-love in her life. She began practicing yoga, taking walks in nature, and making time for creative pursuits like writing and painting. She also started a daily practice of positive self-talk and self-compassion, which helped her to appreciate her own strengths and abilities.

Over time, Sandra found that she had more energy and enthusiasm for life. She was better able to manage stress and anxiety, and felt more confident and self-assured in her interactions with others. By prioritizing her own well-being, Sandra was able to create a more fulfilling and meaningful life for herself and her family.

Meet Ethan, a 28-year-old graphic designer who had been struggling with low self-esteem and negative self-talk for years. Despite his many accomplishments, Ethan found himself constantly comparing himself to others and feeling like he wasn't good enough.

Through self-care practices like exercise and healthy eating, and self-love practices like positive self-talk and self-compassion, Ethan was able to improve his self-esteem and cultivate a greater sense of self-worth. He also began practicing meditation and mindfulness, which helped him to become more present and grounded in the moment.

Over time, Ethan found that he was better able to manage stress and anxiety, and approach challenges with a growth mindset. He was more confident in his own abilities and more accepting of himself and his limitations. By focusing on self-care and self-love, Ethan was able to transform his relationship with himself and create a more positive and fulfilling life.

Sandra and Ethan's stories exemplify the power of self-care and self-love. Sandra's life was transformed as she began prioritizing her well-being by practicing yoga, taking walks in nature, and making time for creative pursuits, while also starting a daily practice of positive self-talk and self-compassion. Ethan improved his self-esteem and cultivated a greater sense of self-worth by practicing self-care practices like exercise and healthy eating, and self-love practices like positive self-talk and self-compassion. He also began practicing meditation and mindfulness, which helped him become more present and grounded in the moment.

As we've been exploring practices for self-care and self-love you can see that they are not selfish acts but rather have numerous benefits for personal growth and well-being. By prioritizing our own needs and well-being and developing a positive relationship with ourselves, we can improve our overall health, reduce stress and anxiety, and cultivate greater self-compassion and self-esteem. You're encouraged to begin implementing these practices into your daily lives and experiencing the benefits of self-care and self-love firsthand.

In this section, we explored the importance of self-awareness and self-love for personal growth and well-being. By practicing self-reflection through journaling, meditation, or quiet contemplation, individuals can become more aware of their inner experiences and develop a deeper understanding of their thoughts, emotions, and behaviors.

We also discussed the significance of identifying limiting beliefs and patterns that may be holding individuals back. By recognizing these beliefs and patterns, individuals can challenge them and create a greater sense of clarity and direction in their lives.

Cultivating self-compassion and positive self-talk is another crucial component of self-reflection and self-love. By treating oneself with kindness, compassion, and understanding, individuals can improve their emotional resilience, increase their self-esteem and confidence, and experience more fulfilling relationships.

Learning to set healthy boundaries and prioritize one's needs is also an essential aspect of self-care and self-love. By doing so, individuals can avoid burnout, reduce stress and anxiety, and gain greater clarity and direction in their lives.

Finally, we explored various practices for self-care and self-love, including exercise, healthy eating, and other forms of self-care. These practices can help individuals improve their physical and mental health, increase their emotional resilience, and experience greater fulfillment and joy in their lives.

Overall, by understanding the importance of self-reflection and self-love, practicing these skills, and incorporating self-care practices into your daily life, one can experience a range of benefits, including increased emotional resilience, greater self-esteem and confidence, and more fulfilling relationships.

To begin incorporating these practices into your life, you are encouraged to start by identifying one area of your life where you would like to cultivate greater self-awareness and self-love. From there, you can use the tips and techniques provided to begin practicing self-reflection and self-love on a regular basis. By making these practices a habit, you can start to experience the benefits of increased self-awareness, self-compassion, and self-esteem in your daily life.

Here are some practical tips and techniques that you can use to implement the practices of self-reflection and self-love in your daily life:

- Journaling: Set aside time each day to reflect on your thoughts and emotions. Write down any patterns or limiting beliefs that you notice and challenge them by reframing them in a more positive light.

- Meditation: Practice mindfulness meditation to increase your awareness of the present moment and improve emotional regulation. Start with just a few minutes each day and gradually increase the amount of time you spend meditating.

- Positive self-talk: Cultivate a more positive internal dialogue by practicing self-compassion and self-acceptance. When negative self-talk arises, challenge it with more positive affirmations and self-talk.

- Identify and challenge limiting beliefs: Identify any beliefs that may be holding you back and challenge them by looking for evidence to the contrary. Reframe negative beliefs in a more positive light.

- Set healthy boundaries: Identify your needs and set healthy boundaries to prioritize your well-being. Learn to say no to commitments that don't align with your goals or values.

- Practice self-care: Make time for activities that you enjoy and that help you recharge. This can include exercise, spending time in nature, or taking a relaxing bath.

In conclusion, cultivating self-reflection and self-love can have a transformative effect on our emotional resilience, self-esteem, and overall well-being. Through the practices we have explored, we can gain greater self-awareness, challenge limiting beliefs, and learn to prioritize our needs and goals. As we move forward, the next section will explore the power of visualization as a tool for goal-setting and achievement. By incorporating techniques for creating vivid and specific mental images of our desired outcomes, and regularly revisiting and updating them, we can stay motivated and focused on the path toward a more fulfilling and purposeful life.

Visualization

INTRODUCTION OVERVIEW: Visualization is a powerful tool that can help individuals achieve their goals and create the life they desire. By using the imagination to create vivid mental images of desired outcomes, individuals can tap into the power of their subconscious mind and align their thoughts, beliefs, and actions with their goals. Visualization has been used by athletes, business leaders, and other successful individuals for decades to achieve peak performance and success. In this section, we will explore the benefits of visualization and provide practical techniques and tips for incorporating it into daily life.

Visualization is a technique that involves creating mental images of desired outcomes, and it has been shown to be a powerful tool for achieving personal and professional goals. Visualization can help individuals to focus their thoughts and beliefs in a positive and productive direction, which can ultimately lead to greater success and achievement.

In this section, we will explore the many benefits of visualization, including increased motivation, improved focus and concentration, and enhanced problem-solving skills. We will also provide practical tips and techniques for incorporating visualization into your daily life, such as creating specific and detailed visualizations, using affirmations to reinforce positive beliefs, and regularly revisiting and updating your visualizations to stay motivated and focused.

One of the primary benefits of visualization is its ability to help individuals set and achieve goals. By creating a clear mental picture of what they want to achieve, individuals can more easily identify the steps they need to take to reach their goals. Visualization can also help individuals to stay motivated and focused, even when faced with obstacles or setbacks.

To incorporate visualization into your daily life, start by setting specific and achievable goals. Once you have identified your goals, take some time to create a detailed mental image of what you want to achieve. Use all of your senses to create a vivid picture of what success looks, sounds, feels, and even smells like.

In addition to creating detailed visualizations, using affirmations can also be an effective way to reinforce positive beliefs and increase motivation. Affirmations are positive statements that are repeated regularly to help reprogram your subconscious mind and reinforce positive beliefs about yourself and your abilities.

Regularly revisiting and updating your visualizations can also be a powerful way to stay motivated and focused. Set aside time each day to review your visualizations and affirmations, and make any necessary updates or revisions to ensure that they continue to reflect your current goals and desires.

Research has shown that visualization can have a positive impact on physical and mental health, as well as overall well-being. For example, a study found that athletes who practiced visualization techniques experienced improved performance and reduced anxiety.

In summary, visualization is a powerful tool that can help individuals to achieve their goals and create the life they desire. By creating specific and detailed mental images of desired outcomes, individuals can tap into the power of their subconscious mind and align their thoughts, beliefs, and actions with their goals. By incorporating visualization techniques into daily life, individuals can improve their motivation, focus, and problem-solving skills, and ultimately achieve greater success and fulfillment.

- **The power of visualization for goal-setting and achievement**

Visualization is a powerful tool for achieving our goals and aspirations. By creating vivid mental images of our desired outcomes, we can tap into the power of our subconscious minds to align our thoughts, beliefs, and actions with our goals. This can help us to overcome obstacles, stay motivated, and ultimately achieve success.

One key aspect of visualization for goal-setting and achievement is the importance of specificity. By creating detailed and specific mental images of what we want to achieve, we can better focus our efforts and actions towards those goals. For example, if we want to get a promotion at work, we can visualize ourselves in the new role, doing the tasks and responsibilities that come with it, and feeling fulfilled and satisfied in our work. This can help us to stay motivated and focused on taking the necessary steps towards that promotion.

Another important aspect of visualization for goal-setting and achievement is the power of emotion. When we visualize our goals, we should aim to engage all our senses and create a strong emotional connection to the outcome we want to achieve. This can help to solidify our commitment to our goals and keep us motivated to take action towards them.

By incorporating visualization into our goal-setting process, we can enhance our ability to achieve our desired outcomes and unlock our full potential. Whether it's a career goal, a health goal, or a personal growth goal, visualization can be a powerful tool for achieving success.

- **Techniques for visualizing vivid and specific images of your desired outcomes**

Visualization is a powerful tool for creating the life you desire, but it is important to create specific and detailed mental images in order to make them more tangible and achievable. In this section, we will explore techniques for visualizing vivid and specific images of your desired outcomes.

One effective technique for creating vivid visualizations is to use all five senses, incorporating details like sounds, smells, and textures to make the image as realistic and tangible as possible. Another technique is to imagine the desired outcome as if it has already happened, creating a sense of certainty and confidence in the mind.

It is important to be clear and specific about what you want to achieve, and to visualize the outcome in as much detail as possible. This can include the people involved, the specific location, and the time frame in which the outcome is desired.

Visualizations can also be enhanced by creating a mental "movie" of the desired outcome, using different camera angles and perspectives to create a multi-dimensional experience. This can help to engage the imagination and create a more immersive visualization.

By using these techniques to create detailed and specific mental images, individuals can enhance the effectiveness of their visualizations and increase the likelihood of achieving their desired outcomes. At the end of this section, we will provide exercises and practical tips for implementing these techniques in your own life.

- **Tips for creating a vision board or other visual representation of your goals**

Creating a vision board or other visual representation of your goals can be a powerful tool for manifesting your dreams and desires. A vision board is a collage of images, words, and phrases that represent the things you want to achieve, and it can be used to help clarify your goals, keep you focused and motivated, and visualize the life you want to create.

To create a vision board, start by gathering images, words, and phrases that resonate with your goals and aspirations. This can include pictures of things you want to own, experiences you want to have, people you want to meet, or accomplishments you want to achieve. You can also include affirmations, quotes, or other inspirational messages that resonate with you.

Once you have gathered your materials, arrange them on a poster board or other surface in a way that feels intuitive and meaningful to you. You can organize your vision board by category, such as career, relationships, health, or personal growth, or you can arrange it in a way that feels visually appealing and inspiring to you.

Once your vision board is complete, display it in a place where you will see it frequently, such as in your bedroom or workspace. Take time each day to look at your vision board and visualize yourself already living the life you desire. Allow yourself to feel the emotions of already having achieved your goals and trust that the Universe is working to bring them to you.

Creating a vision board is just one of the many ways to incorporate visualization into your life. It's a fun and creative way to stay focused on your goals and keep your subconscious mind aligned with your desires. In the next subtopic, we will explore ways to incorporate all five senses into your visualizations to enhance their effectiveness.

- **Incorporating all five senses into your visualizations to enhance their effectiveness**

Visualizing a goal is not just about seeing it in your mind's eye, but also feeling, hearing, smelling, and even tasting it. When you engage all five senses in your visualization, you create a more vivid and compelling experience that is more likely to manifest in reality.

By engaging all of our senses, we can create more vivid and realistic mental images that are more likely to activate the corresponding neural pathways in our brain and generate the emotions associated with our desired outcome, as well as physiological responses. [19, 20, 21] This can help to increase the effectiveness of your visualizations and make them feel more real and tangible.

Let's give it a try. To incorporate all five senses into your visualizations, start by imagining a specific scenario in your mind. It could be a scene from your future, a place you want to visit, or any other situation that represents your desired outcome. Once you have the

Cultivating Mindfulness, Self-Awareness and Growth

scenario in your mind, take a moment to observe it in detail. What do you see? What colors, shapes, and textures are present? Next, think about what you hear in this scenario. Are there any sounds, such as the rustling of leaves, the chirping of birds, or the sound of people talking?

Now, shift your attention to what you can feel in this scenario. Is there a sensation of warmth or coolness? Can you feel the texture of objects in your surroundings? What do you feel physically in your body? Then, pay attention to any scents that may be present in this scenario. Is there a certain smell that you associate with this experience?

Lastly, consider the taste associated with this scenario. What flavors and textures come to mind? Once you've explored each of these senses, try to bring them all together to create a comprehensive and fully immersive visualization.

Take a moment to reflect on what you are feeling after this visualization exercise. Does the scenario feel more real and present to you? Are you more motivated to take action towards your goal? By engaging all of your senses, you can create a powerful and lasting impression that inspires you to take action towards your desired outcome.

As you continue to use this technique, try to pay attention to how your body responds to the different sensory inputs. What emotions do you feel? What physical sensations do you experience? By tuning into your body's response, you can learn to use your senses more effectively in your visualizations and create even more powerful and impactful mental experiences.

- **How to stay motivated and focused by regularly revisiting and updating your visualizations**

To stay motivated and focused on your goals, it is important to regularly revisit and update your visualizations. When we visualize our goals, we create a mental image of what we want to achieve and this image becomes a point of reference that we can use to stay motivated and on track. However, as we progress towards our goals, our desires and priorities may change, so it's important to update our visualizations to align with our current vision.

One technique for staying motivated and focused is to create a routine for revisiting and updating your visualizations. This could be a daily or weekly practice, where you take some time to review your goals and update your mental image of them. During this practice, take the time to fully immerse yourself in your visualization, using all five senses to make it feel as real and tangible as possible.

Another technique is to use your visualizations as a source of inspiration and motivation when you feel stuck or unmotivated. Whenever you're feeling discouraged or unsure of your next steps, take a moment to visualize your desired outcome and remind yourself of why it's important to you. This can help you to reconnect with your goals and rekindle your motivation to take action towards them.

It's also important to be open and flexible with your visualizations, allowing them to evolve and change as your goals and priorities shift. As you progress towards your goals, new opportunities may arise and your desires may change. By regularly revisiting and updating your visualizations, you can ensure that they stay aligned with your current vision and goals.

Staying motivated and focused on your goals is essential for achieving them. Regularly revisiting and updating your visualizations is a powerful technique for staying on track and maintaining your motivation. By creating a routine, using your visualizations as a source of inspiration, and being open to change, you can use this technique to unlock your full potential and achieve your dreams.

In conclusion, visualization is a powerful tool that can help individuals to achieve their goals and create the life they desire. By using the imagination to create vivid mental images of desired outcomes and engaging all five senses, individuals can tap into the power of their subconscious mind and align their thoughts, beliefs, and actions with their goals. In this section, we have explored the benefits of visualization and provided practical techniques and tips for incorporating it into daily life. We have covered topics such as the power of visualization for goal-setting and achievement, techniques for creating specific and detailed visualizations, and how to stay motivated and focused by regularly revisiting and updating your visualizations. Whether you are looking to improve your career, relationships, health, or personal growth, visualization can help you to unlock your full potential and achieve your dreams.

Here are some practical tips and techniques that you can use to implement the practices of visualization in your daily life:

Start with small goals: If you are new to visualization, start with small goals that are achievable in a short period of time. This will help you build confidence and develop your visualization skills.

Use all five senses: Engage all five senses in your visualizations to create a more vivid and compelling experience that is more likely to manifest in reality.

Regularly revisit and update your visualizations: To stay motivated and focused, make sure to regularly revisit and update your visualizations. This will help to reinforce your goals and keep them at the forefront of your mind.

Create a vision board: A vision board is a visual representation of your goals and desires that you can use to inspire and motivate you. It can be created using images, words, and symbols that represent your goals and desires.

Use guided visualization exercises: Guided visualization exercises can be a helpful way to develop your visualization skills and stay motivated. There are many resources available online and in books that provide guided visualization exercises.

By implementing these practical tips and techniques, you can begin to incorporate the power of visualization into your daily life and achieve your goals and desires.

We've explored the power of the imagination to create vivid mental images of desired outcomes and unlock our full potential. In this next section on cultivating healthy relationships, we will explore the impact of our social connections on personal growth and well-being. We will discuss the importance of building healthy relationships through effective communication and conflict resolution skills, developing emotional intelligence through increased self-awareness and empathy, and nurturing supportive relationships with family, friends, mentors, and partners. We will also cover topics such as identifying toxic relationships and setting boundaries, and provide tips for building and maintaining a strong support system. Whether you are looking to improve your personal or professional relationships, or simply build a more fulfilling and supportive social network, this section will provide practical techniques and strategies to help you cultivate healthy and meaningful connections with others.

Cultivating Healthy Relationships (building support system/emotional intelligence)

INTRODUCTION OVERVIEW: The relationships we have with others are critical components of our well-being and personal growth. Healthy relationships can provide support, encouragement, and a sense of belonging, while toxic or negative relationships can cause stress, anxiety, and other mental health issues. In this section, we will explore the importance of cultivating healthy relationships and emotional intelligence as foundational components of personal growth and well-being. We will provide readers with an understanding of the different types of relationships we encounter, how they impact our lives, and practical strategies for building healthy relationships through effective communication, conflict resolution, and boundary-setting. Additionally, we will delve into the concept of emotional intelligence, exploring how this skill can help us manage our own emotions while empathizing with and understanding the emotions of others.

Cultivating healthy relationships is crucial for personal growth and well-being. The people in our lives can have a significant impact on our mental health, self-esteem, and overall happiness. Healthy relationships can provide a sense of belonging, support, and encouragement, while toxic or negative relationships can cause stress, anxiety, and other mental health issues.

In this section, we will explore the different types of relationships we encounter, including romantic relationships, family relationships, friendships, and professional relationships. We'll discuss the impact that these relationships can have on our lives and how to identify signs of unhealthy or toxic relationships.

We will also delve into practical strategies for building healthy relationships, including effective communication, conflict resolution, and boundary-setting. Effective communication is essential for building strong relationships, as it allows us to express our thoughts and feelings while also listening to and understanding the perspectives of others. We will explore different communication styles and provide tips for improving communication in different types of relationships.

Conflict is inevitable in any relationship, but how we handle conflict can make all the difference. We will provide practical strategies for resolving conflicts in a healthy and constructive way, including active listening, compromise, and finding common ground.

Setting boundaries is also a crucial aspect of building healthy relationships. Boundaries help us protect our physical and emotional well-being and communicate our needs and limits to others. We will explore different types of boundaries and provide tips for setting and maintaining healthy boundaries in different types of relationships.

Emotional intelligence is another crucial component of building healthy relationships. Emotional intelligence involves the ability to recognize and manage our own emotions while also empathizing with and understanding the emotions of others. We will explore the different components of emotional intelligence and provide tips for developing this skill, including mindfulness practices, empathy exercises, and self-reflection.

By the end of this section, readers will have a better understanding of how relationships impact personal growth and well-being. They will have gained practical tools and techniques for cultivating healthy relationships through effective communication, conflict resolution, and boundary-setting. Additionally, they will have explored the concept of emotional intelligence and gained tips for developing this skill. With practice and commitment, readers can build a supportive network and develop the skills needed to thrive in all areas of their lives.

- **Understanding the impact of relationships on personal growth and well-being**

Having healthy and supportive relationships is vital for personal growth and overall well-being. Our relationships shape us and influence how we see ourselves, others, and the world around us. Positive relationships can provide emotional support, help us build self-esteem, and give us a sense of belonging. On the other hand, negative relationships can be emotionally draining and cause stress, anxiety, and even physical health problems.

To cultivate healthy relationships, it's important to understand the impact they have on our lives. Positive relationships can help us thrive in many areas of our lives, such as career, health, and personal growth. By having supportive people around us, we can better manage stress, increase our resilience, and stay motivated to achieve our goals. On the other hand, negative relationships can hold us back and make it difficult to reach our full potential.

By understanding the impact of our relationships, we can begin to take steps to nurture the positive ones and set healthy boundaries with the negative ones. Through increased awareness and mindfulness, we can cultivate healthy and meaningful relationships that support our personal growth and well-being.

- **Identifying toxic relationships and setting boundaries**

To cultivate healthy relationships, it is important to be able to recognize and set boundaries with toxic individuals who may be negatively impacting our lives. Identifying toxic relationships can be difficult, as they can manifest in a variety of ways and may not always be obvious. However, by paying attention to how we feel around certain people, we can start to recognize patterns and behaviors that are harmful to our well-being.

When identifying toxic relationships, it is important to pay attention to how we feel around certain individuals. Do we feel drained, anxious, or unhappy after spending time with them? Do they consistently make us feel bad about ourselves or put us down? These are all potential signs of a toxic relationship. It is important to recognize these patterns and to set boundaries with individuals who are negatively impacting our lives.

Setting boundaries is an important part of maintaining healthy relationships. It allows us to communicate our needs and expectations clearly and to prevent others from crossing our boundaries. This can be difficult, particularly if we are used to people-pleasing or have a history of unhealthy relationships. However, by practicing assertiveness and standing up for ourselves, we can create a healthier dynamic in our relationships.

To set boundaries effectively, it is important to be clear about what we will and will not tolerate in our relationships. We should communicate these boundaries clearly and assertively, while also being open to compromise and negotiation. It is also important to enforce these boundaries consistently and to be prepared to step back from relationships that are not healthy or beneficial for us.

By identifying toxic relationships and setting healthy boundaries, we can create space for more positive and fulfilling relationships in our lives. We can build stronger connections with those who support and uplift us, while also protecting our well-being and personal growth. With practice and patience, we can cultivate healthier relationships and build a more positive and supportive network of people around us.

- **Building healthy relationships through effective communication and conflict resolution skills**

Effective communication and conflict resolution skills are essential for building and maintaining healthy relationships. Communication is the foundation of any relationship, and it is through effective communication that we are able to connect with others, express our needs and wants, and resolve conflicts when they arise. When we have healthy communication skills, we are able to build trust and intimacy with others, and establish a foundation for a strong and supportive relationship.

Take the example of Anna and Ron. Anna and Ron had been married for several years, but had been experiencing some difficulties in their relationship. They often argued and struggled to communicate effectively with each other. Through couples therapy, they learned effective communication and conflict resolution skills, including active listening, expressing emotions in a non-threatening way, and taking responsibility for their own part in conflicts. As they started to practice these skills in their relationship, they were able to communicate more effectively, resolve conflicts in a healthier way, and build a stronger and more supportive relationship.

Another example is the story of Manny, who had a difficult time expressing his emotions to his friends and family. He would often become defensive or shut down when conflicts arose, and had a hard time understanding other people's perspectives. Through therapy and self-reflection, he learned effective communication and conflict resolution skills, including identifying and expressing emotions, active listening, and using "I" statements instead of "you" statements. As he started to practice these skills in his relationships, he found that he was able to connect more deeply with others, build stronger and more meaningful relationships, and feel more fulfilled in his personal life.

To build healthy relationships through effective communication and conflict resolution skills, it is important to focus on active listening, expressing emotions in a non-threatening way, and taking responsibility for your own part in conflicts. This includes using "I" statements instead of "you" statements, identifying and expressing emotions, and working towards a resolution that is mutually beneficial for all parties involved. By practicing these skills, we can establish healthy communication patterns and build stronger and more supportive relationships in all areas of our lives.

- **Developing emotional intelligence through increased self-awareness and empathy**

Emotional intelligence is a crucial aspect of cultivating healthy relationships. It involves being aware of and understanding one's own emotions, as well as being able to recognize and empathize with the emotions of others. Developing emotional intelligence requires increased self-awareness and empathy, which can be achieved through various practices and techniques.

One effective way to improve emotional intelligence is through mindfulness meditation. By practicing mindfulness, individuals can increase their self-awareness and become more attuned to their thoughts and emotions. This can help them to better regulate their emotions and respond to situations with greater clarity and compassion.

Another way to develop emotional intelligence is by actively practicing empathy. This involves putting oneself in the shoes of others and understanding their emotions and perspectives. By practicing empathy, individuals can better understand the needs and feelings of others, which can lead to more effective communication and conflict resolution.

In addition, developing emotional intelligence also involves being able to manage one's own emotions and respond to the emotions of others in a healthy and productive way. This can be achieved through practices such as journaling, cognitive-behavioral therapy, and other forms of self-reflection.

For example, let's consider the story of Katherine, who struggled with emotional regulation and often found herself feeling overwhelmed by her emotions. Through regular meditation and journaling, she was able to become more self-aware of her emotions and learn how to manage them more effectively. This helped her to better communicate with her partner and build a stronger and healthier relationship.

Another example is the story of Alex, who found it difficult to empathize with others and often struggled with conflicts in his relationships. Through practicing active listening and empathy, he was able to better understand the perspectives and emotions of others, which led to more effective communication and improved relationships with his loved ones.

In order to develop emotional intelligence and cultivate healthy relationships, it's important to take time to reflect on one's own emotions and learn how to manage them effectively. By practicing mindfulness, empathy, and other forms of self-reflection, individuals can become more attuned to their emotions and better equipped to handle the emotions of others.

- **Nurturing supportive relationships with family, friends, mentors, and partners**

Nurturing supportive relationships with family, friends, mentors, and partners is a crucial aspect of cultivating healthy relationships. Supportive relationships can provide a sense of security, belonging, and validation, which can enhance personal growth and well-being. It is important to be intentional about building and maintaining these relationships in our lives.

One example of nurturing supportive relationships is by practicing active listening. Active listening involves giving your full attention to the person speaking, seeking to understand their perspective and feelings, and responding with empathy and respect. By listening actively, we can deepen our connections with others and show that we care about their thoughts and emotions.

Meet Carla, she had always struggled with building strong relationships. She often felt lonely and isolated, despite having many acquaintances. One day, she decided to take action and actively work on nurturing more supportive relationships. She reached out to a friend she hadn't spoken to in a while and scheduled a coffee date to catch up. During their conversation, Carla listened actively and expressed genuine interest in her friend's life, and in turn, her friend reciprocated. After that initial meeting, Carla made a conscious effort to stay in touch and connect with her friend regularly. Over time, their relationship grew stronger, and Carla felt more supported and less alone. She realized that by showing genuine interest and care for others, and being open to receiving support in return, she could build meaningful and supportive relationships that enhanced her well-being.

Another way to nurture supportive relationships is by being there for your loved ones during difficult times. This involves providing emotional support, whether it's through comforting words, physical touch, or simply being present. By showing up for those we care about, we can strengthen our bonds and foster a sense of trust and reliability.

Ultimately, nurturing supportive relationships requires effort and intentionality. It involves consistently showing up, communicating effectively, and demonstrating empathy and compassion. By doing so, we can create a support system that enriches our lives and helps us to thrive.

- **Tips for building and maintaining a strong support system**

A strong support system is essential for maintaining mental and emotional well-being. By building a network of supportive relationships, individuals can find comfort, guidance, and encouragement during difficult times, as well as celebrate their successes and accomplishments. Here are some tips for building and maintaining a strong support system:

Identify the people in your life who you can count on for support, such as family members, friends, mentors, or coworkers.

Be open and honest with your support system about your needs and feelings, and don't be afraid to ask for help when you need it.

Nurture your relationships by spending quality time with your support system, expressing appreciation, and showing interest in their lives.

Focus on building relationships that are mutually beneficial and positive, and avoid those that are draining or toxic.

Consider joining support groups or online communities that align with your interests or needs, as they can provide a sense of connection and understanding.

Remember that building a support system takes time and effort, but it is a worthwhile investment in your mental and emotional health.

For example, Lara struggled with anxiety and often felt isolated and alone. However, she began to build a support system by joining a support group for individuals with anxiety and making an effort to connect with people who shared similar experiences. By doing so, she found comfort in knowing that she was not alone and gained valuable insights and coping strategies from her support system.

In conclusion, cultivating healthy relationships and emotional intelligence is crucial for personal growth and well-being. In this section, we have explored the impact of relationships on our lives, how to identify toxic relationships and set boundaries, and how to build healthy relationships through effective communication and conflict resolution skills. We have also discussed developing emotional intelligence through increased self-awareness and empathy and nurturing supportive relationships with family, friends, mentors, and partners. Lastly, we provided tips for building and maintaining a strong support system. By implementing these practices, we can create a foundation of healthy relationships and emotional intelligence that will support us throughout our lives.

As we move into the next section on Nutrition and Fitness, we will explore the importance of proper nutrition and exercise for physical and mental health. We will discuss the basics of nutrition and how to build a healthy, balanced diet, as well as tips for incorporating physical activity into our daily routine. We will also explore different types of exercise and strategies for overcoming common obstacles to healthy eating and exercise. By developing healthy habits for long-term success, we can achieve optimal physical and mental health and create a foundation for a fulfilling and vibrant life.

Nutrition and Fitness

INTRODUCTION TO OVERVIEW: The Nutrition and Fitness section of the book emphasizes the importance of good nutrition and regular physical activity in maintaining optimal health and well-being. It provides readers with a comprehensive understanding of the benefits of proper nutrition and exercise, as well as practical tips and strategies for developing healthy habits and overcoming common obstacles.

Proper nutrition and regular physical activity are essential for achieving and maintaining optimal physical and mental health. In this section, we will explore the basics of nutrition, including the importance of macronutrients, micronutrients, and hydration, and how they relate to overall health and well-being. We will also discuss the different types of exercise, including cardio, strength training, and flexibility exercises, and how to incorporate them into your daily routine.

In addition, we will provide practical strategies for overcoming common obstacles to maintaining healthy habits, such as lack of motivation, time constraints, and financial barriers. We will discuss the benefits of developing healthy habits for long-term success and how to stay motivated and accountable to your wellness goals.

By implementing the practices and strategies covered in this section, readers can take control of their health and achieve their wellness goals. Whether you are seeking to lose weight, gain muscle, or simply maintain good health, this section provides actionable tips and techniques for developing healthy habits and maintaining long-term success.

At the end of this section, readers will find exercises and practical tips to help them implement the techniques covered in their daily lives. By engaging with the content and putting these techniques into practice, readers can achieve optimal health and well-being, leading to a happier and more fulfilling life.

- **The importance of proper nutrition and exercise for physical and mental health**

Proper nutrition and exercise are crucial for achieving optimal physical and mental health. Our bodies need a balance of nutrients, vitamins, and minerals to function properly, and regular physical activity helps to strengthen our muscles, improve our cardiovascular health, and boost our mood. In this section, we will explore the importance of nutrition and exercise for overall health and well-being.

Nutrition is the foundation of a healthy lifestyle, and a balanced diet is essential for maintaining good health. We will discuss the basics of nutrition, including the five food groups, recommended daily intakes, and tips for building a healthy, balanced diet. We will also address common misconceptions and myths surrounding nutrition and provide practical tips for making healthy food choices.

Exercise is equally important for physical and mental health. Regular physical activity can help to prevent chronic diseases, improve cardiovascular health, and boost mood and cognitive function. We will provide tips for incorporating physical activity into your daily routine, as well as explore different types of exercise and finding what works best for you.

It's important to understand that nutrition and exercise are interconnected, and proper nutrition is key to fueling your body for physical activity. We will discuss the relationship between nutrition and exercise and how to balance them to achieve optimal health and fitness.

By implementing a healthy lifestyle that includes proper nutrition and exercise, you can improve your physical and mental health, and reduce the risk of chronic diseases. In the next subtopics, we will dive deeper into nutrition and exercise, providing practical tips and techniques for building healthy habits that can lead to long-term success.

- **Understanding the basics of nutrition and how to build a healthy, balanced diet**

Proper nutrition is essential for maintaining good physical and mental health. Understanding the basics of nutrition can help you to build a healthy, balanced diet that provides your body with the nutrients it needs to function optimally.

The foundation of a healthy diet includes a variety of nutrient-dense foods from all of the major food groups, including fruits, vegetables, whole grains, lean proteins, and healthy fats. It is important to select organic foods whenever possible to avoid exposure to harmful pesticides and chemicals. Additionally, avoiding genetically modified organisms (GMOs) is recommended as they can have negative effects on health. These foods provide the body with essential vitamins, minerals, fiber, and other nutrients that are necessary for good health.

As a starting point, a healthy meal plan for a woman might include: breakfast of oatmeal with fresh berries and almonds, a mixed green salad with grilled chicken breast for lunch, and salmon with roasted vegetables for dinner. For a man, a healthy meal plan might include: scrambled eggs with whole-grain toast and avocado for breakfast, a turkey and hummus wrap for lunch, and grilled steak with sweet potato and green beans for dinner.

To build a healthy, balanced diet, it is important to understand the recommended daily intake of each nutrient and how to choose foods that provide them. For example, fruits and vegetables are rich in vitamins, minerals, and fiber, while lean proteins such as chicken, fish, and beans are important sources of protein and other nutrients. Whole grains, such as brown rice and quinoa, provide fiber and essential nutrients, while healthy fats, such as those found in nuts and avocados, are important for brain function and other bodily processes.

Another example of a healthy, balanced meal might include grilled chicken breast with a side of roasted vegetables and a serving of quinoa. This meal provides lean protein, fiber, and essential nutrients from the chicken and vegetables, while the quinoa provides additional fiber and complex carbohydrates for sustained energy.

Following as another example, is sample meal plan for a day for a woman and one for a man, based on a balanced and healthy diet:

For a woman:

Breakfast: 2 boiled eggs, 1 slice of whole-grain toast, 1 small avocado, 1 cup of berries, and 1 cup of coffee or tea

Mid-morning snack: 1 small apple and 1 tablespoon of almond butter

Lunch: Grilled chicken salad with mixed greens, cherry tomatoes, cucumber, red onion, and 1/4 cup of nuts. Dressing: 1 tablespoon of olive oil and 1 tablespoon of balsamic vinegar

Afternoon snack: 1 small container of Greek yogurt and 1/4 cup of berries

Dinner: 4 oz of grilled salmon, 1/2 cup of brown rice, 1 cup of steamed vegetables (e.g. broccoli, carrots, cauliflower), and 1 small sweet potato

For a man:

Breakfast: 3 scrambled eggs, 2 slices of whole-grain toast, 1 small avocado, 1 cup of berries, and 1 cup of coffee or tea

Mid-morning snack: 1 small apple and 2 tablespoons of almond butter

Lunch: Grilled chicken sandwich with whole-grain bread, mixed greens, tomato, avocado, and mustard. Side: 1/2 cup of baby carrots and 1/4 cup of hummus

Afternoon snack: 1 small container of Greek yogurt and 1/2 cup of berries

Dinner: 6 oz of grilled steak, 1/2 cup of quinoa, 1 cup of steamed vegetables (e.g. broccoli, carrots, cauliflower), and 1 small sweet potato

These are just examples and may not be appropriate for everyone. It is important to note that the specific nutrient needs of each individual may vary based on factors such as age, gender, activity level, and overall health status. Consulting with a registered dietitian or healthcare provider can help you to tailor your diet to meet your specific needs and goals.

Throughout the Nutrition and Fitness section, we will continue to explore various topics related to proper nutrition and exercise, including tips for incorporating physical activity into your daily routine, exploring different types of exercise and finding what works for you, and strategies for overcoming common obstacles to healthy eating and exercise. By the end of the section, you will have a comprehensive understanding of how to develop healthy habits for long-term success.

- **Tips for incorporating physical activity into your daily routine**

Regular physical activity is essential for maintaining good health and well-being. Incorporating physical activity into your daily routine can be challenging, especially if you have a busy schedule or are not accustomed to exercise. However, with a little creativity and planning, it is possible to increase your physical activity and reap the benefits of a more active lifestyle.

One way to incorporate physical activity into your daily routine is to find activities that you enjoy and that can easily fit into your schedule. This could include taking a walk during your lunch break, riding your bike to work or school, or doing a quick workout at home. By finding activities that you enjoy and that fit into your schedule, you are more likely to stick with them and make physical activity a regular part of your routine.

Another tip is to start small and gradually increase the intensity and duration of your physical activity. This could include starting with a 10-minute walk and gradually increasing the time and distance each week, or starting with a few simple exercises and gradually building up to a more intense workout. By starting small and gradually increasing the intensity and duration of your physical activity, you can avoid injury and make sustainable progress towards your fitness goals.

It can also be helpful to track your progress and set specific, achievable goals for yourself. This could include tracking the number of steps you take each day, setting a goal to walk or run a certain distance by a specific date, or aiming to complete a certain number of push-ups or other exercises each day. By setting specific, achievable goals and tracking your progress, you can stay motivated and focused on your fitness goals.

Remember, physical activity is not just about the time you spend in the gym or on the track. It can also include everyday activities such as gardening, housework, and playing with your kids or pets. By finding ways to incorporate physical activity into your daily routine, you can improve your physical health, reduce stress, and enhance your overall well-being.

As a specific example, here is a sample of a simple daily exercise routine for a busy working professional:

Cardiovascular exercise and stretching:

10-15 minutes of stretching and warm-up exercises in the morning

A brisk 20-minute walk during lunch break

10 minutes of resistance band exercises in the evening

Cardiovascular exercise and strength training:

30-minute jog or bike ride in the morning

A 15-minute bodyweight workout during lunch break

20-minute weightlifting session in the evening

Remember, these are just examples and should be tailored to your individual needs and preferences. The key is to find physical activities that you enjoy and that fit into your schedule, and to gradually increase the intensity and duration of your activity over time.

- **Exploring different types of exercise and finding what works for you**

Regular exercise can have numerous benefits for both physical and mental health, including improved cardiovascular function, increased muscle strength and endurance, and reduced risk of chronic disease. There are many different types of exercises that can be incorporated into a fitness routine, including cardio, strength training, and flexibility exercises. Let's explore further into different types and their benefits.

Cardio exercises are important for improving cardiovascular health and burning calories. These can include activities such as walking, running, cycling, swimming, or group fitness classes such as dance, kickboxing, or indoor cycling.

Strength training exercises are essential for building muscle mass and increasing metabolism. These can include exercises such as weight-lifting, bodyweight exercises, or resistance band exercises. Examples include squats, lunges, push-ups, pull-ups, and bicep curls.

Flexibility exercises are important for maintaining range of motion and reducing the risk of injury. These can include stretching exercises, yoga, or Pilates. Examples include downward dog, warrior pose, and spinal twists.

To get the most benefit from exercise, it's important to incorporate a variety of different exercises into your routine. This can help to challenge different muscle groups, prevent boredom, and reduce the risk of overuse injuries. Additionally, it's important to progress your workouts over time, gradually increasing the intensity, duration, or weight lifted as your fitness level improves.

Here are some examples of exercises that can be incorporated into a well-rounded fitness routine:

Walking: A low-impact exercise that can be done anywhere, walking can help to improve cardiovascular health, strengthen leg muscles, and burn calories.

Squats: A strength training exercise that targets the legs and glutes, squats can be done with or without weights and can help to improve lower body strength and tone.

Yoga: A form of flexibility exercise that also incorporates strength and balance training, yoga can help to improve flexibility, reduce stress, and promote overall well-being.

High-Intensity Interval Training (HIIT): A cardio exercise that involves short bursts of intense activity followed by periods of rest, HIIT can help to improve cardiovascular health, burn calories, and boost metabolism.

Resistance Band Rows: A strength training exercise that targets the upper back and shoulders, resistance band rows can be done with a resistance band and can help to improve posture and upper body strength.

By incorporating a variety of exercises into your routine, you can create a well-rounded fitness program that supports overall health and well-being. Remember to consult with a healthcare professional before starting any new exercise program, and start slowly and gradually increase the intensity and duration over time.

- **Strategies for overcoming common obstacles to healthy eating and exercise**

Here, we will provide practical tips and strategies to help readers overcome common barriers to healthy eating and exercise, so they can achieve their goals and improve their overall health and wellbeing.

One of the most common obstacles to healthy eating is lack of time. Many people feel that they don't have enough time to plan and prepare healthy meals, and end up relying on convenience foods that are often high in calories, sugar, and fat. To overcome this obstacle, it's important to prioritize your health and make time for meal planning and preparation. This could include setting aside a few hours each week to prepare healthy meals in advance, or investing in a meal delivery service that provides healthy, pre-made meals.

Another common obstacle to healthy eating is budget constraints. Healthy foods can often be more expensive than their less healthy counterparts, which can make it difficult to stick to a healthy eating plan. To overcome this obstacle, consider shopping for fresh, seasonal produce at local farmers' markets or purchasing frozen fruits and vegetables, which can be less expensive than fresh produce. Additionally, it can be helpful to plan your meals and make a shopping list in advance to avoid impulse purchases that can add up quickly.

When it comes to exercise, lack of motivation is a common barrier. Many people struggle to stay motivated and stick to an exercise routine, particularly when they don't see immediate results. To overcome this obstacle, it's important to find activities that you enjoy and that fit into your schedule, whether that's taking a dance class, going for a walk with a friend, or practicing yoga at home. Additionally, setting small, achievable goals and tracking your progress can help to boost motivation and keep you on track.

Another common obstacle to exercise is physical limitations or injuries. It's important to listen to your body and avoid exercises that cause pain or discomfort. Instead, focus on low-impact activities, such as swimming, cycling, or using an elliptical machine, that are easier on the joints and can still provide a great workout. It may also be helpful to work with a physical therapist or personal trainer to develop a customized exercise plan that takes into account any physical limitations or injuries.

In addition to these strategies, it's important to remember that overcoming obstacles to healthy eating and exercise is a process, and it may take time and effort to make lasting changes. It can be helpful to enlist the support of family and friends, or to seek the guidance of a registered dietitian or personal trainer who can provide additional motivation and accountability.

Remember, the key to overcoming common obstacles to healthy eating and exercise is to stay focused on your goals, prioritize your health, and make small, sustainable changes that can add up to big results over time.

- **Developing healthy habits for long-term success**

Developing healthy habits is crucial to achieving and maintaining good nutrition and fitness, and it requires consistency and commitment. One way to develop healthy habits is to start small and gradually increase your efforts. It's important to set realistic goals and track your progress to help you stay motivated.

Another key to developing healthy habits is to make it a part of your daily routine. This can be done by scheduling exercise at the same time every day, meal prepping healthy food for the week, or taking a walk during your lunch break. It's also important to find an accountability partner, whether it's a friend, family member, or personal trainer, to help keep you on track and motivated.

In addition to setting realistic goals and incorporating healthy habits into your daily routine, it's important to recognize and overcome common obstacles to healthy eating and exercise. Some of these obstacles may include lack of time, access to healthy food, and social pressures. It's important to have strategies in place to overcome these obstacles, such as finding healthy meal options at fast-food restaurants or making time for exercise by waking up earlier or finding small windows of time throughout the day.

Overall, developing healthy habits for long-term success is a crucial component of good nutrition and fitness. By setting realistic goals, making healthy habits a part of your daily routine, and finding ways to overcome obstacles, you can make lasting changes in your lifestyle and achieve optimal health and wellness.

In conclusion, this section on Nutrition and Fitness has emphasized the importance of proper nutrition and physical activity for overall health and wellness. By understanding the basics of nutrition, incorporating physical activity into your daily routine, and developing healthy habits for long-term success, you can achieve your health and wellness goals. These practices are not only important for physical health, but also for mental and emotional well-being, as they can help reduce stress, improve mood, and increase self-confidence. By implementing the tips and strategies discussed in this section, you can build a strong foundation for a healthy and fulfilling life.

Developing a growth mindset and resilience

INTRODUCTORY OVERVIEW: Developing a growth mindset and resilience are essential for personal growth and success. A growth mindset is the belief that our abilities and qualities can be developed through dedication and hard work. This mindset promotes a love of learning and a willingness to embrace challenges and setbacks as opportunities for growth. On the other hand, a fixed mindset is the belief that our abilities and qualities are fixed and cannot be changed.

In this section, we will explore the power of having a growth mindset and building resilience. We will begin by discussing the differences between a fixed and growth mindset, and why having a growth mindset is critical for personal and professional growth. We will also explore how to develop a growth mindset and resilience, with practical strategies for overcoming obstacles and setbacks.

Cultivating Mindfulness, Self-Awareness and Growth

One of the ways to build resilience is through self-care, creating a supportive network, and developing positive self-talk. We will delve into each of these strategies, discussing how to practice self-care, create a supportive network, and engage in positive self-talk. Additionally, we will discuss the fear of failure, which can hold us back from taking risks and pursuing our goals. We will provide tips and techniques for overcoming this fear and developing a growth mindset through risk-taking.

Finally, we will discuss the importance of celebrating progress and successes along the way. We'll provide practical techniques and tips for tracking progress, setting achievable goals, and celebrating small wins. By taking the time to recognize and appreciate our successes, we can build momentum and stay motivated on the path towards our long-term goals.

By the end of this section, you will have a comprehensive understanding of how to cultivate a growth mindset and build resilience. With practical tips and exercises, you will be able to incorporate these strategies into your daily life and overcome obstacles and setbacks with a positive attitude. Developing a growth mindset and resilience can lead to a more fulfilling and meaningful life, and we encourage you to engage with the content, reflect on your own mindset and resilience, and start implementing the strategies discussed in this section.

- **Understanding the difference between a fixed and growth mindset**

Developing a growth mindset involves understanding the difference between a fixed and growth mindset. Individuals with a fixed mindset believe that their qualities, skills, and abilities are predetermined and unchangeable. In contrast, those with a growth mindset believe that their skills and abilities can be developed through hard work, learning, and dedication.

For example, someone with a fixed mindset may believe that they are not a "math person" and will never be able to improve their math skills. On the other hand, someone with a growth mindset recognizes that while they may not be naturally skilled in math, they can improve their abilities through practice, learning, and persistence.

Recognizing the benefits of a growth mindset for personal and professional growth is also an important aspect of this subtopic. By embracing a growth mindset, individuals can increase their resilience, motivation, and sense of self-efficacy. They can also become more open to learning and feedback, which can lead to greater success and achievement.

As an example, someone who has a growth mindset may view challenges and setbacks as opportunities for growth and development, while someone with a fixed mindset may view them as signs of their innate limitations and give up easily.

In order to develop a growth mindset and overcome obstacles and setbacks with resilience, it's important to have effective strategies in place. This can include practicing positive self-talk, building a strong support system, and engaging in self-care activities that promote physical and emotional well-being.

As an example, someone who faces a setback may choose to engage in activities that they enjoy and that help them to relax, such as taking a yoga class or spending time with friends. They may also practice positive self-talk, reminding themselves of their strengths and past successes, and seeking support from loved ones.

Navigating the fear of failure and developing a growth mindset through risk-taking is another important aspect of this subtopic. By taking calculated risks and stepping outside of their comfort zone, individuals can develop greater resilience, self-confidence, and adaptability.

For example, someone who has a fear of public speaking may challenge themselves to give a speech at a local event or volunteer to lead a meeting at work. By taking these risks and pushing themselves outside of their comfort zone, they can develop greater confidence and a sense of personal growth.

Finally, celebrating progress and successes along the way is an important aspect of developing a growth mindset. By recognizing and celebrating small wins and accomplishments, individuals can build momentum and motivation towards achieving their goals.

Someone who has set a goal of running a 5K may celebrate their progress by completing a 1K run or achieving a personal best time in training. By celebrating these small successes, they can build motivation and confidence towards achieving their ultimate goal.

I hope these scenarios were helpful. Overall, developing a growth mindset and resilience is essential for personal and professional growth. By recognizing the benefits of a growth mindset, embracing effective strategies, and celebrating progress and successes, individuals can unlock their full potential and achieve their dreams.

- **Recognizing the benefits of a growth mindset for personal and professional growth**

A growth mindset is the belief that our abilities and intelligence can be developed through dedication and hard work. In contrast, a fixed mindset is the belief that our abilities are set in stone and cannot be changed. Recognizing the benefits of a growth mindset can have a significant impact on our personal and professional growth.

Individuals with a growth mindset tend to approach challenges with a positive attitude and view failures as opportunities for growth and learning. This can lead to increased motivation, resilience, and perseverance in the face of obstacles. Additionally, having a growth mindset can lead to increased creativity and innovation, as individuals are more willing to take risks and try new things.

To cultivate a growth mindset, it's important to practice self-reflection and awareness of our thought patterns. Recognize when negative self-talk or limiting beliefs are holding you back, and challenge them with positive affirmations and a willingness to learn and improve. Seek out opportunities for growth and learning, and surround yourself with others who share your values and are committed to personal and professional development.

For example, imagine a person who is hesitant to take on a new project at work because they don't feel confident in their abilities. With a fixed mindset, this person might think "I'm just not good at this kind of work, so there's no point in even trying." But with a growth mindset, they might think "This is a great opportunity for me to learn and develop new skills, and even if I don't succeed right away, I can use this experience to grow and improve for the future."

By recognizing the benefits of a growth mindset and cultivating it in our daily lives, we can open ourselves up to new opportunities and achieve greater personal and professional success.

- **Strategies for overcoming obstacles and setbacks with resilience**

Developing a growth mindset requires resilience and the ability to bounce back from setbacks and challenges. In fact, setbacks and challenges can be valuable opportunities for growth and development if we approach them with the right mindset. By adopting a growth mindset, we can reframe obstacles as opportunities to learn and grow, rather than insurmountable barriers.

To build resilience and overcome obstacles, it's important to start by recognizing our internal self-talk and the messages we give ourselves when we face setbacks. Instead of giving into negative self-talk and limiting beliefs, we can choose to reframe the situation and focus on the possibilities for growth and development. This may involve acknowledging and accepting the emotions that arise when we face setbacks, but also choosing to shift our focus to the lessons we can learn from the experience.

Another important strategy for building resilience is to seek out support and connection with others. Building a strong support system of friends, family, mentors, and colleagues can provide us with the encouragement, motivation, and perspective we need to overcome obstacles and keep moving forward. Additionally, connecting with others who have faced similar challenges can be empowering and validating.

Self-care is also essential for building resilience and overcoming obstacles. Taking care of our physical, emotional, and mental health through regular exercise, healthy eating, mindfulness practices, and restful sleep can provide us with the energy and clarity we need to tackle challenges and setbacks.

Finally, it's important to celebrate progress and successes along the way, even if they may seem small at first. By recognizing and celebrating our growth and development, we can build the confidence and resilience we need to continue moving forward and overcome future obstacles.

Here's an example of how these strategies can be applied in practice:

John had been working hard to launch his own business, but had hit several setbacks along the way. He had experienced funding challenges, encountered unexpected competition, and struggled with self-doubt and limiting beliefs. However, he decided to approach these challenges with a growth mindset, seeing them as opportunities to learn and improve his business model.

He began to shift his self-talk, reminding himself of his goals and focusing on the lessons he was learning from each setback. He also reached out to his mentor and fellow entrepreneurs for support and perspective, gaining valuable advice and encouragement.

Additionally, John made self-care a priority, incorporating daily exercise and mindfulness practices into his routine. He celebrated even small successes along the way, such as securing a new client or making progress on his business plan.

Through these strategies, John was able to build resilience and overcome the obstacles he had faced, ultimately launching a successful business that was built on the lessons he had learned from his setbacks.

- **Tips for building resilience through self-care, support systems, and positive self-talk**

One of the most important ways to build resilience is through self-care. This means taking care of your physical, mental, and emotional health on a regular basis. This can include getting enough sleep, eating a healthy diet, engaging in regular exercise, and taking time to do things that you enjoy. Self-care can help to reduce stress, boost your mood, and increase your overall well-being, making it easier to navigate difficult situations with greater ease.

Another important strategy for building resilience is to build strong support systems. This means surrounding yourself with people who are supportive and encouraging, and who can help you through challenging times. Your support system can include friends, family members, mentors, or professional colleagues. It's important to have people you can turn to for help and guidance when you need it, and who can offer a listening ear and a shoulder to lean on when things get tough.

Positive self-talk is also an important aspect of building resilience. This means talking to yourself in a positive and encouraging way, even during difficult times. Instead of focusing on negative thoughts or self-doubt, try to focus on your strengths and abilities, and remind yourself that you are capable of overcoming any challenge. By using positive self-talk, you can build a greater sense of confidence and self-assurance, which can help you to overcome obstacles and setbacks more easily.

Overall, building resilience is essential for personal and professional growth, and can help you to navigate challenging situations with greater ease and confidence. By practicing self-care, building strong support systems, and using positive self-talk, you can cultivate a growth mindset and build the resilience you need to achieve your goals and overcome obstacles.

- **Navigating fear of failure and developing a growth mindset through risk-taking**

Everyone experiences fear of failure at some point in their lives. Whether it's a new job opportunity, a personal project, or a big decision, the fear of failure can be paralyzing and prevent us from taking risks that could lead to personal and professional growth. However, by developing a growth mindset, we can learn to embrace failure as a necessary part of the learning process and use it as an opportunity to learn and grow.

To navigate the fear of failure, it's important to start by reframing our mindset. Instead of seeing failure as something to be avoided, try to view it as a stepping stone towards success. Remember that failure is a natural part of the learning process and that every successful person has experienced failure in some form.

Next, start taking small risks to build up your confidence and develop your resilience. This could mean trying something new or unfamiliar, speaking up in a meeting, or asking for feedback on a project. By taking small steps, you can gradually build up your comfort level with risk-taking and learn to push past the fear of failure.

It's also important to have a supportive network of friends, family, or colleagues who can offer encouragement and help you stay motivated. Surround yourself with people who believe in your potential and who can offer constructive feedback and support as you navigate challenges and setbacks.

Remember, developing a growth mindset and overcoming the fear of failure is not a one-time event, but a continuous journey. Be patient with yourself and celebrate the small successes along the way. By embracing risk-taking and learning from failure, you can develop the resilience and confidence needed to achieve your personal and professional goals.

So, don't let fear hold you back from pursuing your dreams. Embrace the challenges, take risks, and believe in your ability to learn and grow from failure. With a growth mindset, anything is possible.

- **Celebrating progress and successes along the way**

When we focus on our goals and the things we want to achieve, it can be easy to overlook the progress we've made along the way. However, recognizing and celebrating our successes, no matter how small they may seem, is essential for maintaining motivation and momentum towards our goals.

One effective strategy for celebrating progress and successes is to break down our goals into smaller, more achievable milestones. This allows us to celebrate each step along the way, rather than only focusing on the final outcome. We can also use a journal or other tracking method to record our progress and acknowledge the hard work we've put in.

It's important to also take time to acknowledge and appreciate the hard work and effort we've put in, even if we haven't achieved our end goal yet. Celebrating small victories can help to keep us motivated and build confidence in our abilities. By focusing on the positive aspects of our journey, we can create a positive feedback loop that helps to drive us towards our goals.

Real-world examples of celebrating successes and achievements include throwing a small party or gathering with friends and family, treating ourselves to a special meal or activity, or simply taking a moment to reflect on the progress we've made and giving ourselves a pat on the back.

Remember, even the smallest victories are worth celebrating. By celebrating our progress and successes along the way, we can maintain motivation, build confidence, and ultimately achieve our goals.

In this section on "Developing a Growth Mindset and Resilience", we've explored the difference between fixed and growth mindsets, recognized the benefits of a growth mindset, learned strategies for overcoming obstacles and setbacks with resilience, and discovered tips for building resilience through self-care, support systems, and positive self-talk. We've also explored the importance of celebrating progress and successes along the way. By developing a growth mindset and building resilience, we can navigate challenges with greater ease and achieve our goals with greater confidence. In the next section, we will explore the importance of developing a positive self-image and cultivating self-love for improved mental health and well-being.

In this section, we explored the importance of cultivating healthy relationships through building a support system and developing emotional intelligence. We also discussed the crucial role that nutrition and exercise play in physical and mental health. As we move into our next section, Creating healthy habits and self-care, we will delve into the importance of self-care for overall health and well-being. We will explore strategies for creating healthy habits in nutrition, exercise, sleep, and other areas, as well as tips for overcoming resistance to change and building new habits. Additionally, we will discuss the importance of developing a self-care routine that works for you and your lifestyle, and explore different types of self-care practices such as mindfulness, relaxation, and self-compassion. By incorporating these practices into our daily lives, we can build a foundation for long-term health and well-being.

Creating healthy habits and self-care

INTRODUCTION OVERVIEW: In today's fast-paced world, it's easy to get caught up in the hustle and bustle of everyday life and neglect our physical, mental, and emotional well-being. But by creating healthy habits and practicing self-care, we can prioritize our own needs and ensure that we are functioning at our best. In this section, we will explore the importance of self-care and creating healthy habits, and provide practical tips and techniques for incorporating them into our daily lives.

We will cover various topics, such as the benefits of self-care for physical and mental health, the different types of self-care practices and how to prioritize them, creating and maintaining healthy habits in different areas of life such as diet, exercise, sleep, and relaxation, and developing a self-care routine that works for us.

By implementing the strategies and techniques covered in this section, we can improve our overall well-being, increase our energy, reduce stress, and improve our relationships with others. This section serves as a guide for readers to develop a personalized self-care plan and maintain healthy habits for long-term success.

At the end of the book, readers will find a series of exercises that they can use to reflect on their own experiences and apply the concepts learned in each section to their own lives. These exercises are intended to help readers apply the knowledge gained in the book and develop a personalized plan for personal growth and well-being.

- **The importance of self-care for overall health and well-being**

Self-care is a crucial component of maintaining our physical, mental, and emotional health. It involves taking intentional and consistent actions to prioritize our own needs and well-being, and it is essential for preventing burnout, stress, and other negative health outcomes. Self-care looks different for everyone, and it can include activities such as exercise, meditation, reading, spending time with loved ones, and many other practices that bring us joy and relaxation.

It is important to recognize that self-care is not a luxury or an indulgence, but rather a necessity for maintaining optimal health and well-being. Taking care of ourselves allows us to better manage stress, reduce the risk of chronic illness, and improve our relationships and overall quality of life. By prioritizing self-care, we can also become more productive, focused, and motivated in our personal and professional lives.

However, self-care can be challenging for many people, particularly those who struggle with feelings of guilt or self-doubt about taking time for themselves. It's important to remember that taking care of yourself is not selfish, but rather a responsible and necessary act of self-preservation. By prioritizing self-care and making it a regular part of our routine, we can improve our overall health and well-being and become more resilient and empowered individuals.

- **Identifying and prioritizing your self-care needs and activities**

Self-care is an essential aspect of overall health and well-being, and it involves identifying and prioritizing your individual needs and activities. The first step in this process is to become aware of the different areas of your life that require attention and care, including physical, emotional, mental, and spiritual well-being. Once you have identified these areas, you can start to explore the specific self-care activities and practices that can support and nourish each one.

It's important to note that self-care is not a one-size-fits-all approach, as everyone has unique needs and preferences. For some, self-care may involve engaging in physical activity, while for others, it may mean spending time alone in nature or practicing mindfulness meditation. The key is to identify the activities that work best for you and to make them a regular part of your routine.

One effective way to prioritize your self-care needs and activities is to create a self-care plan. This plan can help you stay on track with your self-care goals and ensure that you are making time for the activities that are most important to you. To create a self-care plan, start by setting specific goals and identifying the actions that will help you achieve them. It can be helpful to break your goals down into smaller, more manageable steps and to schedule specific times in your calendar for your self-care activities.

Overall, identifying and prioritizing your self-care needs and activities can have a positive impact on your physical, emotional, and mental well-being. By taking care of yourself, you can improve your overall quality of life, reduce stress and anxiety, and develop a greater sense of resilience and inner strength.

- **Strategies for creating healthy habits in nutrition, exercise, sleep, and other areas**

Creating healthy habits is essential for maintaining a balanced and fulfilling lifestyle. Whether it's improving your nutrition, starting an exercise routine, or getting enough sleep, building healthy habits takes time, effort, and commitment. To successfully create new habits, it's important to start with small, achievable goals and gradually build on them.

One strategy is to use the "habit loop" model, which consists of a cue, routine, and reward. The cue is the trigger that initiates the behavior, the routine is the behavior itself, and the reward is the positive outcome that reinforces the behavior. By identifying the cues and rewards associated with a behavior, you can modify the routine and make it easier to establish new habits.

Another helpful strategy is to use the power of positive self-talk and visualization. By using affirmations, such as "I am capable of making healthy choices," and visualizing yourself successfully achieving your goals, you can reinforce positive habits and overcome self-doubt or negative self-talk.

For example, if your goal is to improve your nutrition, start with small changes such as adding more fruits and vegetables to your meals, reducing your sugar intake, or drinking more water. As you begin to see positive results and feel more confident in your ability to make healthy choices, you can gradually incorporate more changes into your diet.

In addition to nutrition, exercise is also an important aspect of building healthy habits. Find an exercise routine that works for you and start with small, achievable goals such as walking for 30 minutes a day or taking a fitness class once a week. As you begin to see the benefits of regular exercise, you can gradually increase the intensity and frequency of your workouts.

Finally, getting enough sleep is crucial for overall health and well-being. Develop a regular sleep routine by going to bed and waking up at the same time each day, avoiding caffeine and electronic devices before bedtime, and creating a comfortable sleep environment. By prioritizing your sleep and establishing a routine, you can improve your overall health and energy levels.

By implementing these strategies and gradually building healthy habits, you can improve your physical and mental well-being and enjoy a more balanced and fulfilling lifestyle.

Next, we will discuss tips for overcoming resistance to change and building new habits.

- **Tips for overcoming resistance to change and building new habits**

When it comes to building healthy habits and self-care routines, one of the biggest challenges people face is resistance to change. Breaking old habits and creating new ones can be difficult and uncomfortable, even if we know that it's for our own benefit. To overcome resistance and build new habits, it's important to start with small, manageable changes and build on them gradually over time.

One helpful strategy is to set specific, measurable goals for yourself, and track your progress towards them. This can help you stay motivated and focused, and give you a sense of accomplishment as you see yourself making progress towards your goals. It's also important to celebrate your successes along the way, no matter how small they may seem.

Another effective technique is to identify and challenge any negative self-talk or limiting beliefs that may be holding you back. Our thoughts and beliefs can have a powerful impact on our behavior, and it's important to cultivate a growth mindset that allows for change and progress. Instead of focusing on past failures or perceived limitations, focus on the possibilities for growth and improvement.

It's also helpful to find accountability and support in the form of a friend, family member, or professional who can help you stay on track and provide encouragement and motivation. Having someone to share your goals and progress with can help to keep you accountable and motivated, and provide a sense of community and support.

Remember, building new habits and overcoming resistance to change takes time and effort, but the rewards of improved health and well-being are well worth it. By starting small, setting specific goals, challenging negative self-talk, and finding support and accountability, you can create lasting changes and a healthier, more fulfilling life.

In the next subtopic, we will explore how to develop a self-care routine that works for you and your lifestyle, and the benefits that self-care can bring to your overall health and well-being.

- **Developing a self-care routine that works for you and your lifestyle**

Developing a self-care routine that works for you and your lifestyle is essential for maintaining a healthy and balanced life. Self-care is not just about treating yourself to a spa day or a bubble bath, but it also includes creating a consistent routine that prioritizes your physical, mental, and emotional needs.

To develop a self-care routine, start by identifying the activities and practices that make you feel good, calm, and balanced. This could be anything from yoga, meditation, or taking a walk in nature, to reading a book, listening to music, or simply taking a nap. Experiment with different practices and take note of how they make you feel.

It's important to find a balance between activities that are relaxing and those that are energizing. Relaxing activities, such as taking a bath, can help you unwind and de-stress, while energizing activities, such as going for a run, can help boost your energy levels and improve your mood.

In addition to incorporating self-care activities into your routine, it's important to make time for healthy habits such as proper nutrition, exercise, and sleep. By consistently making time for these activities, you can create a self-care routine that supports your overall health and well-being.

Remember, developing a self-care routine is a personal process, and what works for one person may not work for another. It's important to be flexible and willing to adapt your routine to fit your changing needs and lifestyle.

By prioritizing your self-care needs and consistently practicing healthy habits, you can create a more balanced and fulfilling life that supports your physical, mental, and emotional health.

Some examples of self-care routines may include waking up early to meditate or exercise, setting aside time each day to read or journal, taking a walk during your lunch break, or winding down before bed with a relaxing activity such as stretching or practicing gratitude.

Remember, self-care is not a luxury, but a necessity for maintaining a healthy and balanced life. By making self-care a priority and developing a routine that works for you, you can improve your overall well-being and better manage stress and challenges in your life.

- **Exploring different types of self-care practices, such as mindfulness, relaxation, and self-compassion**

Self-care is crucial for maintaining overall health and well-being, and exploring different self-care practices can help you find what works best for you. Some examples of self-care practices include mindfulness, relaxation techniques, and self-compassion.

Mindfulness involves paying attention to the present moment, without judgment or distraction. Mindfulness meditation is a popular form of mindfulness practice, but you can also incorporate mindfulness into everyday activities, such as eating, walking, or even brushing your teeth. By practicing mindfulness, you can improve your focus, reduce stress and anxiety, and increase your overall sense of well-being.

Relaxation techniques, such as deep breathing, progressive muscle relaxation, and guided imagery, can also be effective in reducing stress and promoting relaxation. By learning and practicing relaxation techniques, you can improve your ability to manage stress and achieve a more relaxed and peaceful state of mind.

Self-compassion is another important self-care practice that involves treating yourself with kindness, empathy, and understanding, particularly in times of difficulty or failure. By practicing self-compassion, you can increase your resilience, reduce feelings of shame or self-criticism, and improve your overall sense of self-worth.

By exploring these different types of self-care practices, you can find the ones that work best for you and make them a regular part of your self-care routine. This can help you to improve your overall health and well-being, and better manage stress and difficult emotions.

It's important to remember that self-care is not a luxury, but a necessity for maintaining our physical and mental health. By prioritizing self-care practices and incorporating them into our daily lives, we can better manage stress and improve our overall well-being.

We must be diligent in our self-care practices, as they can help us to be more resilient and adaptable in the face of adversity. In the next section, we will be exploring the benefits of meditation and mindfulness for reducing stress and increasing well-being, which can also play an important role in our self-care practices.

In conclusion, we have explored the importance of self-care for our overall health and well-being, as well as strategies for creating healthy habits in nutrition, exercise, sleep, and other areas. We have learned tips for overcoming resistance to change and building new habits, as well as different types of self-care practices, such as mindfulness, relaxation, and self-compassion.

By prioritizing our self-care needs and establishing healthy habits, we can improve our physical, mental, and emotional well-being, and live a more fulfilling life. I encourage you to explore the different self-care practices and strategies that we have discussed and find what works best for you.

In the next section, we will delve into the benefits of meditation and mindfulness for reducing stress and increasing well-being. We will explore various meditation techniques, tips for establishing a regular practice, and strategies for managing thoughts and emotions during meditation and throughout the day. So, let's dive in and learn how to cultivate mindfulness in our daily lives.

Meditation/Mindfulness

INTRODUCTION STATEMENT: Meditation and mindfulness are practices that can help individuals achieve a greater sense of inner peace, calm, and mental clarity. In this section, we will explore the benefits of meditation and mindfulness, as well as provide practical guidance and tips for incorporating these practices into your daily life.

We will start by defining what meditation and mindfulness are, and how they differ from one another. We will also explore the various forms of meditation, such as mindfulness meditation, guided meditation, and loving-kindness meditation, and provide tips for selecting the form that best suits your needs.

We will then dive into the benefits of meditation and mindfulness, including improved mental and emotional health, stress reduction, increased focus and concentration, and greater self-awareness. We will also discuss how mindfulness can be applied to other areas of life, such as relationships and work.

In addition to discussing the benefits of meditation and mindfulness, we will also provide practical techniques and strategies for incorporating these practices into your daily life. We will cover topics such as creating a dedicated meditation space, developing a regular meditation routine, and managing thoughts and emotions during meditation and throughout the day.

Finally, we will discuss the importance of self-compassion and non-judgment in the practice of meditation and mindfulness, and how these qualities can be nurtured through the practice of loving-kindness meditation.

As the final chapter of the book, the section on meditation and mindfulness offers readers a powerful tool for promoting inner peace and well-being. With the techniques and strategies provided in this section, readers will be equipped to develop a regular meditation and mindfulness practice, and reap the many benefits that these practices offer.

The book concludes with "7 Exercises for Living a More Fulfilling Life," which provides readers with practical exercises that correspond to each of the seven sections of the book, as well as an additional exercise for cultivating gratitude. These exercises offer readers the opportunity to put into practice the strategies and techniques they have learned throughout the book, and to deepen their personal growth and well-being.

- **Understanding the benefits of meditation and mindfulness for reducing stress and increasing well-being**

Meditation and mindfulness have been shown to have a variety of benefits for reducing stress and increasing overall well-being. These practices can help individuals manage their emotions, reduce anxiety, and improve their ability to focus and concentrate.

One of the key benefits of meditation and mindfulness is stress reduction. When individuals practice mindfulness, they learn to be present in the moment and observe their thoughts and emotions without judgment. This can help reduce anxiety and stress levels, as individuals are better able to recognize and manage their negative thoughts and emotions.

In addition to stress reduction, meditation and mindfulness have been linked to increased emotional regulation and improved mental health. Studies have shown that these practices can help individuals with depression, anxiety, and post-traumatic stress disorder (PTSD) by reducing symptoms and improving overall well-being. [22, 23, 24, 25]

Meditation and mindfulness can also help individuals improve their ability to focus and concentrate. By training the mind to be present in the moment and focus on a particular task, individuals can improve their cognitive performance and increase their productivity. This can be especially beneficial in professional settings or when studying for exams.

Other potential benefits of meditation and mindfulness include improved sleep quality, increased self-awareness and empathy, and even physical health benefits such as lower blood pressure and reduced inflammation.

It's important to note that these benefits may not be immediate, and that regular practice is necessary to see long-term results. However, the benefits of meditation and mindfulness can be profound and far-reaching, making them a valuable addition to any individual's self-care routine.

In the next sections of this book, we will explore different techniques for incorporating mindfulness into everyday activities, different types of meditation practices, such as mindfulness meditation, guided meditation, and loving-kindness meditation, tips for establishing a regular meditation practice, strategies for managing thoughts and emotions during meditation and throughout the day, and ways to incorporate mindfulness into other areas of life, such as relationships and work.

- **Techniques for incorporating mindfulness into everyday activities**

Meditation and mindfulness are powerful tools for reducing stress and promoting overall well-being. In addition to formal meditation practices, incorporating mindfulness into everyday activities can provide numerous benefits. By bringing attention to the present moment and fully engaging in routine activities, we can cultivate a sense of calm and focus that can carry over into all areas of our lives.

Techniques for incorporating mindfulness into everyday activities can include simple practices such as washing dishes mindfully, brushing teeth mindfully, or even driving mindfully. By fully engaging in these routine activities and bringing our awareness to the present moment, we can reduce stress and improve our overall well-being.

There are several different types of meditation practices that can be explored, including mindfulness meditation, guided meditation, and loving-kindness meditation. Each type of meditation practice offers unique benefits and applications, such as developing greater awareness, increasing compassion, or managing difficult emotions.

Establishing a regular meditation practice can be challenging, but it is important for experiencing the full benefits of meditation and mindfulness. By setting aside a consistent time and space for meditation, we can establish a routine and make it a regular part of our day.

Managing thoughts and emotions during meditation and throughout the day is an important aspect of mindfulness practice. Techniques such as observing thoughts without judgment and practicing self-compassion can help us to stay present and focused, even when difficult emotions arise.

Finally, bringing mindfulness into other areas of life, such as relationships and work, can further enhance the benefits of mindfulness practice. By cultivating greater awareness and compassion in all areas of our lives, we can improve our well-being and the well-being of those around us.

- **Exploring different types of meditation practices, such as mindfulness meditation, guided meditation, and loving-kindness meditation**

Meditation is a practice that has been used for centuries to cultivate inner peace and a sense of well-being. There are many different types of meditation, each with its own unique benefits and techniques. In this subtopic, we will explore several different types of meditation practices, including mindfulness meditation, guided meditation, and loving-kindness meditation.

Mindfulness meditation is one of the most well-known and widely practiced types of meditation. It involves focusing your attention on the present moment and observing your thoughts and feelings without judgment. This type of meditation can help reduce stress, increase self-awareness, and improve concentration and focus. To practice mindfulness meditation, find a quiet place to sit and focus on your breath. When your mind wanders, simply bring it back to your breath without judgment.

Guided meditation is a form of meditation that is often used for relaxation and stress reduction. It involves listening to a recorded voice that guides you through a meditation practice. Guided meditations can be customized for specific needs, such as reducing anxiety, improving sleep, or enhancing creativity. They can also be practiced individually or in a group setting.

Loving-kindness meditation, also known as Metta meditation, is a type of meditation that focuses on cultivating feelings of love and compassion toward yourself and others. This practice involves silently repeating phrases of love and well-being, such as "May I be happy" or "May you be at peace." Loving-kindness meditation can help increase feelings of empathy, reduce feelings of isolation, and promote positive emotions.

Exploring different types of meditation practices can help you find a style that works best for your individual needs and preferences. Whether you prefer to practice alone or in a group, with a guided recording or in silence, there is a type of meditation that can benefit you. By incorporating meditation into your daily routine, you can reduce stress, improve your overall well-being, and increase your ability to manage difficult emotions and situations.

One way to practice mindfulness meditation is to follow these steps:

1. Find a quiet and comfortable place to sit. This could be a cushion on the floor, a chair, or even a park bench. Close your eyes or keep them slightly open, and begin to focus your attention on your breath.

2. Notice the sensation of the air moving in and out of your nostrils, the rise and fall of your chest, or the expansion and contraction of your belly. Whenever your mind begins to wander, gently bring it back to the sensation of your breath.

3. As you continue to focus on your breath, you may notice other thoughts, emotions, or physical sensations arise. Acknowledge these without judgment, but don't get caught up in them. Simply observe them and return your focus to your breath.

4. You can set a timer for your meditation practice, starting with just a few minutes and gradually building up to longer periods. Some people find it helpful to use a guided meditation app or recording to provide structure and support for their practice.

5. Remember that meditation is a practice, not a performance. It's natural for your mind to wander, and you may have days where it feels particularly challenging to stay focused. Be patient with yourself, and keep coming back to the practice. Over time, you may notice a greater sense of calm, clarity, and emotional well-being in your daily life.

In the next subtopic, we will discuss tips for establishing a regular meditation practice, as well as strategies for managing thoughts and emotions during meditation and throughout the day.

- **Tips for establishing a regular meditation practice**

Meditation can be a powerful tool for reducing stress and improving overall well-being, but many people struggle to establish a regular practice. However, by incorporating a few key tips, it's possible to make meditation a consistent part of your daily routine.

One of the most important things to do when establishing a meditation practice is to set aside a specific time and space for your practice. This can help to create a sense of routine and make it easier to prioritize your practice. It's also important to start with short sessions and gradually increase the length of your meditation practice over time.

Another tip for establishing a regular meditation practice is to find a meditation style that works for you. There are many different types of meditation, including mindfulness meditation, guided meditation, and loving-kindness meditation, and each style has its own unique benefits. Experimenting with different styles can help you find one that resonates with you and makes it easier to stick with your practice.

Consistency is key when it comes to building a meditation practice, so it's important to make meditation a non-negotiable part of your daily routine. You can also try to incorporate mindfulness into other areas of your life, such as during daily activities or while on a walk.

Ultimately, establishing a regular meditation practice takes time and patience, but the benefits of a consistent practice can be transformative. By setting aside time each day to quiet your mind and connect with your inner self, you can cultivate greater calm, clarity, and presence in your life.

- **Strategies for managing thoughts and emotions during meditation and throughout the day**

Managing our thoughts and emotions is a crucial aspect of meditation and mindfulness practice, as well as our overall well-being. Here are some strategies that can help:

Acknowledge and accept your thoughts and emotions: Instead of trying to push away or ignore your thoughts and emotions, acknowledge them and accept them as a natural part of the human experience. This can help to reduce the intensity of negative emotions and prevent them from building up and causing further stress.

Practice non-judgmental awareness: When meditating or simply going about your day, try to observe your thoughts and emotions without judgment or criticism. This can help to reduce the power of negative self-talk and increase your ability to respond to situations in a calm and rational way.

Cultivate self-compassion: Treat yourself with the same kindness and compassion you would offer to a friend going through a difficult time. Recognize that it's okay to make mistakes and that self-improvement is a process, not a destination.

Use mindfulness techniques to refocus your mind: When your mind starts to wander or get caught up in negative thoughts, use mindfulness techniques such as focusing on your breath or body sensations to bring your attention back to the present moment.

Practice relaxation techniques: Incorporating relaxation techniques such as progressive muscle relaxation or deep breathing exercises into your daily routine can help to reduce stress and increase feelings of calm and well-being.

Let's look to Jake for example of how strategies for managing thoughts and emotions during meditation and throughout the day can be helpful:

Jake had been struggling with anxiety and negative thoughts for a while, which had been affecting his work and personal life. He decided to give mindfulness meditation a try, but found that he couldn't keep his mind from wandering, and his negative thoughts were overwhelming him.

He sought guidance from a meditation teacher who helped him understand that it's normal for thoughts to arise during meditation, and that the practice is about observing them without judgment and allowing them to pass. Jake also learned different techniques to focus his attention and calm his mind, such as breathing exercises and visualization.

As Jake began incorporating mindfulness meditation into his daily routine, he noticed that his negative thoughts and anxiety became more manageable. He also started applying the same strategies throughout the day, such as taking deep breaths and taking a break when he felt overwhelmed.

Through consistent practice, Jake developed the ability to observe his thoughts and emotions with more detachment, which helped him make more rational decisions and respond to situations more calmly. He also found that he was able to enjoy his relationships and daily activities more fully.

In summary, the strategies for managing thoughts and emotions during meditation and throughout the day can have a transformative effect on one's well-being, and can help individuals develop greater emotional resilience and inner peace.

By incorporating these strategies into your daily routine, you can develop a greater sense of self-awareness and emotional regulation, both during meditation and throughout the day.

It's important to remember that managing thoughts and emotions is a skill that takes practice and patience. Be kind and patient with yourself as you work to develop these strategies, and don't be afraid to seek support from a therapist or mental health professional if needed.

Overall, the ability to manage thoughts and emotions is an important aspect of our well-being, and practicing mindfulness and meditation can help to develop this skill. By incorporating these strategies into our daily lives, we can learn to respond to challenging situations in a more calm and centered way, ultimately leading to greater happiness and fulfillment.

- **Incorporating mindfulness into other areas of life, such as relationships and work**

We must first recognize the importance of mindfulness in all aspects of our lives. Mindfulness is not just a practice that we engage in for a few minutes each day; it is a way of being that can transform the way we relate to ourselves and others, and can help us navigate the ups and downs of life with greater ease and resilience.

Throughout this book, we have discussed various techniques and practices for cultivating mindfulness, and in this final subtopic, we will explore how we can take the principles of mindfulness off the cushion and into our daily lives. By incorporating mindfulness into our relationships, our work, and all areas of our lives, we can experience greater peace, happiness, and fulfillment.

To illustrate the power of incorporating mindfulness into other areas of life, let me share my own story. For many years, I struggled with feelings of stress and overwhelm in my professional life. I often felt like I was constantly behind and could never catch up, and my relationships with colleagues and clients suffered as a result.

Through practicing mindfulness and learning to apply its principles in my work, I was able to shift my mindset and approach to my work. I learned to focus on the present moment, to prioritize my tasks, and to let go of unnecessary distractions and worries. As a result, I was able to increase my productivity, improve the quality of my work, and enhance my relationships with my colleagues and clients.

Let's explore strategies for incorporating mindfulness into other areas of life, such as relationships and work, and we will provide tips and guidance for how to apply mindfulness in practical ways that can make a real difference in our lives.

Incorporating mindfulness into different aspects of life, such as relationships and work, is a natural progression once you have started to establish a regular mindfulness practice. Mindfulness can help improve communication, empathy, and emotional regulation, which are all important components of healthy relationships.

One way to incorporate mindfulness into relationships is to actively listen and be present during conversations. When you're talking with someone, try to focus all of your attention on what they're saying without getting distracted by your own thoughts or the environment around you. This will help you fully understand their perspective and respond more thoughtfully.

Mindfulness can also be applied to the workplace to reduce stress and improve focus. Taking a few minutes throughout the day to practice mindfulness can help you stay centered and grounded, even in the face of challenging or stressful situations. Mindfulness can also help you increase your productivity and focus by allowing you to be fully present and engaged in your work.

Another way to incorporate mindfulness into your work is to set boundaries and take breaks. This can help you avoid burnout and maintain a healthy work-life balance. When you take breaks, try to do something that is mindful and rejuvenating, such as going for a walk or practicing yoga.

Incorporating mindfulness into all areas of your life can help you cultivate greater awareness, emotional regulation, and empathy. By being present in the moment, you can improve your relationships, increase your productivity, and reduce stress and burnout.

For example, one of the participants in our mindfulness workshop, Sarah, had been struggling with work-related stress and difficulty communicating with her colleagues. Through mindfulness practice, Sarah was able to cultivate greater awareness and empathy, which improved her communication and allowed her to better navigate challenging situations at work. Additionally, Sarah began to prioritize self-care and set boundaries, which helped her maintain a healthier work-life balance and reduce stress.

Overall, incorporating mindfulness into other areas of life beyond formal meditation can help you live a more mindful and fulfilling life.

By incorporating mindfulness into all areas of your life, you can create a more balanced, fulfilling, and mindful way of living. It may take time and practice, but the benefits are well worth it.

As we conclude, I want to provide you with a helpful resource to continue your journey towards personal growth and well-being. Throughout the book, we've explored various topics, from self-reflection and self-love to developing a growth mindset, and from cultivating healthy relationships to incorporating mindfulness into everyday life.

In each section, I've provided valuable insights and strategies to help you on your journey, and now, I want to offer you practical techniques that you can use to continue implementing these ideas in your life. The following pages will provide you with specific tips, exercises, and practices for each of the seven sections covered in the book.

It's my hope that these techniques will help you to further develop your self-awareness, overcome limiting beliefs, build stronger relationships, and establish healthy habits and practices that support your overall well-being. I encourage you to try out as many of the techniques as you'd like and find the ones that work best for you. Remember, the key to personal growth is consistency and dedication, and I believe these practical techniques will help you along that journey.

I want to thank you for taking this journey with me, and I wish you all the best on your path to greater well-being.

Conclusion

Congratulations on completing "Cultivating Mindfulness, Self-Awareness and Growth: 7 Exercises for Living a More Fulfilling Life"! As we come to the end of this book, I want to take a moment to reflect on the journey that we have taken together. The 7 exercises presented in this book were carefully crafted to guide you towards a more fulfilling life, and I hope that you have found them helpful in your personal growth and self-discovery journey.

I want to remind you that personal growth is a lifelong process, and the exercises in this book are just a starting point. It's important to continue to practice self-reflection, mindfulness, and self-care to maintain your well-being and continue to evolve and transform yourself. The Evolutionary Body System, the program that inspired this book, is based on the idea that we are all capable of evolving and transforming ourselves, regardless of our age or life circumstances. The techniques presented in this book are the same practices that I have used to transform my life, and I am honored to share them with you.

As you continue on your journey, keep in mind the importance of setting clear goals, cultivating healthy relationships, and developing a growth mindset. Remember that obstacles, setbacks, and adversity are a natural part of our life journey, and it's important to approach them with resilience and a positive attitude.

I encourage you to continue exploring and experimenting with the exercises in this book, as well as incorporating other practices that resonate with you. Remember that everyone's journey is unique, and it's important to find what works for you and your individual needs.

Thank you for taking the time to read "Cultivating Mindfulness, Self-Awareness and Growth: 7 Exercises for Living a More Fulfilling Life". I hope that it has been a valuable resource for you on your journey towards a more fulfilling life. Remember to stay present, continue learning, and keep growing!

7 Exercises for Living a More Fulfilling Life

Congratulations on reaching the final section of the book! These exercises have been carefully crafted in sequence to guide you on a journey towards a more fulfilling life. Each section builds upon the previous one, providing you with practical exercises to implement the knowledge and techniques learned throughout the book.

The order of the sections was chosen to create a path of least resistance, starting with self-reflection and self-love to help you develop a positive relationship with yourself, which is the foundation for all other growth. From there, we move on to visualization, which helps you identify and set clear goals for yourself. We then explore building healthy relationships and emotional intelligence, which is crucial for overall well-being.

Next, we dive into nutrition and fitness, which are vital for physical and mental health, followed by developing a growth mindset and resilience, which will help you overcome obstacles and setbacks. Then, we focus on creating healthy habits and self-care, which is essential for maintaining balance and overall health.

Finally, we end with meditation and mindfulness, which ties all of these practices together and helps you cultivate a greater sense of self-awareness and mindfulness. This final exercise provides a powerful tool for greater self-awareness and overall well-being.

These exercises are designed to help you integrate all of these practices into your daily life for greater overall well-being.

7 Exercises for Living a More Fulfilling Life

Here are some practical techniques to implement for each section:

Self-reflection and self-love:

1. Set aside time each day for self-reflection and introspection

2. Practice gratitude by writing down things you are thankful for each day

3. Start a journal and write down your thoughts and feelings

4. Take time for yourself to relax and unwind

5. Use positive affirmations to cultivate self-compassion and positive self-talk

6. Prioritize your needs and set healthy boundaries

Visualization:

1. Create a vision board to visualize your goals

2. Visualize specific outcomes in vivid detail, using all five senses

3. Regularly revisit and update your visualizations to stay motivated and focused

4. Write down your goals and affirmations to keep them at the forefront of your mind

5. Use visualization to reduce stress and anxiety

Cultivating Healthy Relationships:

1. Practice effective communication skills, such as active listening and "I" statements

2. Set boundaries and say "no" when necessary

3. Surround yourself with positive and supportive people

4. Express gratitude and appreciation to those who support and uplift you

5. Practice empathy and emotional intelligence

6. Foster healthy relationships through trust, respect, and open communication

Nutrition and Fitness:

1. Plan out your meals and snacks in advance

2. Incorporate a variety of nutrient-dense foods into your diet

3. Choose whole, unprocessed foods whenever possible

4. Make exercise a regular part of your routine

5. Find an exercise routine that you enjoy and stick to it

6. Set achievable fitness goals and track your progress

Developing a Growth Mindset and Resilience:

1. Practice self-compassion and positive self-talk

2. Embrace challenges and view them as opportunities for growth

3. Celebrate progress and successes along the way

4. Seek support and build a strong support system

5. Use visualization and mindfulness techniques to overcome obstacles

6. Take calculated risks and learn from failure

Creating Healthy Habits and Self-Care:

1. Identify your self-care needs and make time for them in your schedule

2. Develop a healthy sleep routine and prioritize adequate rest

3. Incorporate mindfulness practices into your daily routine

4. Start small and gradually build healthy habits over time

5. Use positive affirmations to cultivate a sense of self-love and self-worth

6. Surround yourself with people who support and uplift you

Meditation/Mindfulness:

1. Set aside time each day for meditation or mindfulness practice

2. Practice deep breathing and relaxation techniques

3. Use mindfulness to manage stress and anxiety throughout the day

4. Incorporate mindfulness into other areas of your life, such as work and relationships

5. Explore different types of meditation, such as guided meditation or loving-kindness meditation

6. Join a meditation group or take a class to deepen your practice

7. These are just a few practical techniques for each section. Remember, everyone's journey is unique, and it's important to find what works best for you.

Acknowledgments

I would like to express my deepest gratitude to all those who supported and encouraged me on this journey. Your unwavering belief in me and my work has been a source of inspiration and motivation. Your presence in my life has made this endeavor all the more meaningful, and I am truly grateful for your ongoing support.

To the readers of this book, I extend my heartfelt thanks for your interest and encouragement. It is my sincere hope that the exercises and practices presented in this book will bring positive transformations in your life and help you achieve greater fulfillment and well-being.

Thank you all from the bottom of my heart.

References and Web Links

1. Asghar, Dr. Andleeb (n.d.). The science of self-love: The evidence based benefits of loving yourself. Ness Labs. Retrieved from https://nesslabs.com/self-love

2. Eurich, Tasha (2018, January 4). What self-awareness really is (and how to cultivate it). Retrieved from https://hbr.org/2018/01/what-self-awareness-really-is-and-how-to-cultivate-it

3. Eichenseher, Tasha (2022, April 21). How to Develop Self-awareness and Why it's Important. Medically reviewed by Bethany Juby, PsyD. PsychCentral. Retrieved from https://psychcentral.com/health/self-awareness

4. Sandoiu, A. (2018, March 23). Why self love is important and how to cultivate it. Medical News Today. Retrieved from https://www.medicalnewstoday.com/articles/321309

5. Goldsmith Turow, Rachel (2023, May 8). Mindfulness meditation and self-compassion: A clinical psychologist explains how these science-backed practices can improve mental health. MedicalXpress. Retrieved from https://medicalxpress.com/news/2023-05-

mindfulness-meditation-self-compassiona-clinical-psychologist.html

6. Goldsmith Turow, Rachel (2023, May 5). Mindfulness meditation and self-compassion: A clinical psychologist explains how these science-backed practices can improve mental health. The Conversation. Retrieved from https://theconversation.com/mindfulness-meditation-and-self-compassion-a-clinical-psychologist-explains-how-these-science-backed-practices-can-improve-mental-health-198731

7. Goldsmith Turow, Rachel (2023, May 5). Mental health: Mindfulness meditation and self-compassion. PhillyVoice. Retrieved from https://www.phillyvoice.com/mental-health-mindfulness-meditation-self-compassion/

8. Goldsmith Turow, Rachel (2022, December 30). Self-compassion shows more mental benefit than mindfulness. Psychology Today. Retrieved from https://www.psychologytoday.com/us/blog/self-talk-science/202212/self-compassion-shows-more-mental-benefit-than-mindfulness

9. Calmer. (2020, December 16). How to practice self-reflection. Retrieved from https://www.thisiscalmer.com/blog/how-to-practise-self-reflection

10. Gupta, S. (2023, May 26). The importance of self-reflection: How looking inward can improve your mental health. Verywell Mind. Retrieved from https://www.verywellmind.com/self-reflection-importance-benefits-and-strategies-7500858

11. Davis, T. (2019, October 7). What is self-reflection and why it matters for wellness. Psychology Today. Retrieved from https://www.psychologytoday.com/us/blog/click-here-happiness/201910/what-is-self-reflection-and-why-it-matters-wellness

12. Cherry, Kendra (2022, August 10). What is Cognitive Behavioral Therapy (CBT)?. Medically reviewed by Rachel Goldman Ph.D., FTOS. Verywell Mind. Retrieved from https://www.verywellmind.com/what-is-cognitive-behavior-therapy-2795747

13. Mayo Clinic. (2019). Cognitive behavioral therapy. In Mayo Clinic Family Health Book (5th ed.). Retrieved from https://www.mayoclinic.org/tests-procedures/cognitive-behavioral-therapy/about/pac-20384610

14. Holland, Kimberly and Nave, Katie (2022, April 27). Cognitive Behavioral Therapy for Depression: How Does It Work? Healthline. Retrieved from https://www.healthline.com/health/depression/cognitive-behavioral-therapy

15. Wells, Katie (2019, July 31). Talking to Yourself With Self-Compassion & Why it's Healthy. Wellness Mama. Retrieved from https://wellnessmama.com/mindset/self-compassion/

16. Ruggeri, Christine (2020, July 10). How to Practice Positive Self Talk for Health and Happiness. DrAxe.com. Retrieved from https://draxe.com/health/positive-self-talk/

17. Riopel, Leslie (2019, June 2). 15 Most Interesting Self-Compassion Research Findings. PositivePsychology.com. Retrieved from https://positivepsychology.com/self-compassion-research/

18. Coelho, S., & Smith, J. (2022, September 7). The Benefits of Self-Compassion. PsychCentral.com. Medically reviewed by Danielle Wade, LCSW. Retrieved from https://psychcentral.com/blog/practicing-self-compassion-when-you-have-a-mental-illness

19. Bailey, Regina (2019, July 16). Overview of the Five Senses. ThoughtCo. Retrieved from https://www.thoughtco.com/five-senses-and-how-they-work-3888470

20. Rago, Rebecca (2014, October 9). Emotion and Our Senses. Tufts University, Emotion, Brain & Behavior Laboratory. Retrieved from https://sites.tufts.edu/emotiononthebrain/2014/10/09/emotion-and-our-senses/

21. Bradford, Alina (2023, January 31). The Five and More Human Senses. Live Science. Retrieved from https://www.livescience.com/60752-human-senses.html

22. Swaim, E. (2022, April 20). Meditation May Improve PTSD Symptoms — Here's How to Try It. Healthline. Medically reviewed by Cheryl Crumpler, PhD. Retrieved from https://www.healthline.com/health/mental-health/ptsd-meditation

23. US Dept of Veterans Affairs PTSD: National Center for PTSD. (n.d.). Mindfulness Practice in the Treatment of Traumatic Stress. Retrieved from https://www.ptsd.va.gov/gethelp/mindfulness_tx.asp

24. Ferguson, S. (n.d.). Tips for meditating when you have PTSD. Headspace. Retrieved from https://www.headspace.com/articles/meditating-with-ptsd

25. NIH National Center for Complementary and Integrative Health. (2020, March). Mind and Body Approaches for Stress and Anxiety: What the Science Says. Retrieved from https://www.nccih.nih.gov/health/providers/digest/mind-and-body-approaches-for-stress-science

Yolanda Trevino

Cultivating Mindfulness, Self-Awareness and Growth

Yolanda Trevino